VITAMINS
Their Use and Abuse

VITAMINS
Their Use and Abuse

Joseph V. Levy, Ph.D.

&

Paul Bach-y-Rita, M.D.

LIVERIGHT 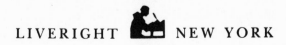 NEW YORK

FIRST EDITION

Library of Congress Cataloging in Publication Data

Levy, Joseph Victor, 1928–
      Vitamins : their use and abuse.
      Bibliography: p.
      Includes index.
      1. Vitamin therapy. 2. Vitamins in human
nutrition. 3. Avitaminosis. I. Bach-y-Rita,
Paul, joint author. II. Title. DNLM: 1. Vitamins—
Therapeutic use. 2. Vitamins—Adverse effects.
QU160 L668v
RM259.L49   1976   612'.399   75-44347
ISBN 0-87140-616-0

1 2 3 4 5 6 7 8 9 0

Contents

Preface

The fact that individuals continue to consume vitamins in amounts greatly exceeding recommended minimum allowances for good health probably reflects in part the lack of confidence in the authorities in the nutrition establishment who assert what is "minimum" and what is "good health." On the other hand, many individuals consume what appear to be unnecessary amounts of vitamins because of: (a) vitamin hucksterism in the marketplace, (b) wide publication of nutritional fads, (c) advocacy of miraculous prophylactic or therapeutic effects of vitamins, (d) physicians specifically prescribing vitamins, (e) anecdotal accounts of vitamin benefits from other lay persons, (f) empirical observations that a certain vitamin restored "vigor," "sexual drive," "endurance," "better eyesight," etc., or (g) any combination of the above reasons.

True vitamin deficiencies are acknowledged to result from (1) inadequate dietary intake, (2) poor absorption or utilization of vitamins, (3) increased excretion, (4) increased requirements (for example, in certain disease states). Responsible nutritionists, scientists, and physicians agree that for normal persons in good health consumption of a well-balanced diet provides all the necessary vitamins, and vitamin deficiencies will not occur.

Even though a balanced diet may provide most of the vitamin needs of normal, healthy adults, a number of special situations may require supplementing the diet with additional vitamins. These include pregnancy, infancy, old age, certain genetic conditions, several disease states, malnutrition, inadequate diet because of weight reduction or religious reasons, the use of certain medicines, vigorous exercise, inclusion in the diet of some vitamin-destroying foods, and a sunless climate.

Most of the special situations listed require medical advice regarding vitamin supplementation. In many of these situations, the necessary vitamins are used as medicines. We certainly do not recommend self-medication. For example, a person with pernicious anemia who treated himself with folic acid might appear healthy in the short run but might be covering up the development of neurological damage due to a Vitamin B_{12} deficiency. Self-medication may also lead to excessive vitamin intake and toxicity (see Glossary). Since it is logical to assume that altered biochemical reactions precede clinical signs of the vitamin deficiency, it follows that only tests of specific metabolic functions would reveal the precise vitamin deficiency. It is advisable to leave these decisions to a physician. Thus, the information presented in this book is for general orientation only, and is not intended for self-diagnosis or treatment.

Some brief examples may illustrate some complex vitamin needs: Normal pregnancy makes heavy vitamin demands both for the mother and for the fetus, and abnormal pregnancies may produce exceptional vitamin demands. For example, abnormal Vitamin B_6 metabolism may be related to toxemia of pregnancy, since substances related to Vitamin B_6 are handled quite differently by pregnant women. Infants, especially when formula fed, usually require vitamin supplements. Furthermore, the vitamins are more rapidly depleted and thus infants have a much smaller safety margin. Rare genetic vitamin deficiency problems may be present, and these may be difficult to diagnose.

Numerous disease states require vitamin supplementation, either because of the primary disease (such as malnutrition and genetic vitamin deficiencies), or due to the destruction of vitamins by the medicines taken to alleviate the disease. For example, the long-term use of barbiturates produces a marked decrease in blood levels of Vitamin D, and thus adult epileptics taking such drugs should receive ten times the theoretical basal requirement of Vitamin D. The use of penicillamine, such as in Wilson's disease or in heavy metal poisoning, interferes with Vitamin B_6

metabolism. Isoniazid, a drug used to treat tuberculosis, can produce detrimental effects on nerves that can usually be prevented by Vitamin B_6. Other drugs can act as antimetabolites and produce vitamin deficiencies. Second degree malnutrition due to loss of appetite or inability to take a variety of food may also lead to relative vitamin deficiencies.

Some foods contain vitamin-destroying factors. For example, a large intake of raw egg whites can produce biotin (see Glossary) deficiencies, with symptoms that include loss of appetite, muscle pains, and dry, scaly skin. Raw fish and clams contain an enzyme, thiaminase, which can split thiamine (see Glossary). This enzyme does not seem to produce human vitamin deficiencies, but is important to cattle raising, since it is found in certain plants and ferns and can produce a vitamin deficiency in cattle known as Bracken's Disease.

Many of these special situations will be discussed in greater detail in this book. Yet for the person with none of these vitamin deficiencies the question remains—Should I take vitamins? The authors, in their personal and professional lives, have been impressed with the confusion, conflicting information, controversy, and claim and counterclaim existing in the field of vitaminology (the science of vitamins). It occurred to us that there was a real need to clarify the situation for the general public.

We live in an era of consumerism. It is no longer sufficient to advise "Buyer Beware." It is wiser to "know your product" or "check the claims." These are the necessary passwords to understanding the mass of materials we are exposed to daily concerning health issues such as the use of vitamins.

It was because of this need to bridge the gap between the scientific lore of vitamins and the layperson's need for knowledge and assistance that we undertook to write this book.

Our objective is simple: When the reader is finished with this book, he or she will be better equipped to question and understand his or her needs for vitamins, and what they do and do not do in the body. Thus, we hope the reader will be able to critically evaluate the many claims from the manufacturers and others who hold vested (although not necessarily commercial) interests or

positions on vitamin use and particularly to evaluate current vitamin topics that are under intense debate and scrutiny. We have
approached our objective by critically reviewing and evaluating
the scientific literature on vitamins. This we have done from the
point of view of general biomedical scientists. However, our review has been selective. We did not intend to survey every aspect
of vitamins. We promote no magic cures or panaceas. We seek
only to inform, and add to the reader's knowledge about a complicated subject that interests us all.

The authors wish to acknowledge the keen and thoughtful
manuscript review and editing provided by Marsha and Eileen
Bach-y-Rita. Their astute comments and observations early in
our writing aided in the formulation of several topics covered in
these pages. We also wish to thank Mr. Robert Bowen for his
stimulating remarks that focussed our appreciation on the need
for a scientific yet non-textbook discussion of vitamins. We
greatly appreciate the typing skills of Suzanne Schafer, who prepared several drafts of our manuscript.

I

VITAMINS IN DAILY LIFE

What Is a Vitamin?

It is not easy to define vitamins. For example, Dr. Karl Folkers (see Primary Sources) has called them organic nutritional substances present in low concentration in the body. They are natural components of enzyme systems required for normal cellular activity. Vitamins may thus catalyze (i.e., facilitate or enhance) required cellular reactions occurring in the body. They may be derived externally from the body (e.g., by diet or by administration of the pure substance by mouth or injection), or they may be made by the body from natural bodily reactions. Thus, Vitamin D may be produced by the body by the action of sunlight upon some basic tissue constituent such as cholesterol or ergosterol. Similarly, Vitamin B_{12} may be formed from the metabolic activity of certain microorganisms in the gastrointestinal tract.

Based upon such definitions, some substances that are commonly called "vitamins" might be reclassified. Vitamin A might be considered a hormone rather than a vitamin. Dr. Folkers and his associates may prefer not to classify Vitamin E as a true vitamin within their definition. On the other hand, many substances are being called "vitamins" without the rudimentary evidence that they should be so designated. The essential nutrients called free fatty acids are sometimes referred to as "Vitamin F." Substances derived from citrus extracts (called bioflavanoids [see Glossary]) are often designated "Vitamin P" since they allegedly are important in maintaining normal capillary (small blood vessel) permeability. Many substances have been called vitamins on far less evidence than this.

Is there not some official, government-regulated set of rules and guidelines for allowing a substance to be called a vitamin, or promoted as such? Surprisingly, the answer is no. For example, The U.S. Food and Drug Administration, which is charged with the responsibility of regulating claims that can be made for drugs and other substances under their jurisdiction, does not have an official, legally recognized definition of a vitamin. This surprises many people. However, the FDA, through its appropriate divisions, does monitor and question the promiscuous or unjustified claims of promoters of substances that are being sold to consumers as vitamins. Thus, while the FDA may not have an official, legally sanctioned definition of a vitamin, it has taken cases to court to prohibit the substances being so promoted from being called "vitamins." Based upon expert scientific testimony, many of these cases are won by the FDA, since the scientific consensus is that the substance under question does not fulfill the commonly accepted definition or criteria for a vitamin. However, because of loose or vague criteria often used for defining "vitamin," various promoters, faddists, and groups continue to call their favorite substance a vitamin. Since the layman has no precise definition, when he hears the term "vitamin" being applied to some substance, he assumes that everyone has agreed upon this designation. This is not true, of course.

It thus appears that the scientific community, the federal agencies that regulate foods and drugs (and the claims made for them), and the consumer may have to tolerate wide variations and impressions as to what actually may be called a "vitamin."

At the least, we can say that vitamins are organic substances that are ordinarily found in our diets. They are distinct from other essential nutrients such as proteins, fats, carbohydrates, minerals. In small amounts, usually in the milligram range, they are generally effective in preventing diseases (or correcting illnesses). (Vitamin B_{12} is effective in the microgram level, i.e., one-millionth of a gram.)

Historically, the first use of the word "vitamine" was by Casmin Funk. He used this term because he thought the substances were *amines* (nitrogen-containing substances) essential to life *(vita)*. Of course, we now know that all vitamins are not amines. Nonetheless, his original term has persisted.

Vitamins are conveniently divided into two chemical classes: The fat-soluble vitamins, such as vitamins A, D, E, and K, and the water-soluble vitamins that include the B vitamins and Vitamin C. These categories are of great importance since the properties of being fat soluble or water soluble influence the way in which the vitamins are absorbed and distributed in body tissues and how long they persist in the body. For example, the fat-soluble vitamins, such as A and D, are accumulated in the fatty structures of the body and are not rapidly cleared by the body. Continued and heavy consumption of such vitamins may lead to excessive tissue accumulation of these substances, with the result that toxicity may develop. This is a medically serious problem called hypervitaminosis. (*Hyper* means excessive or great, *vitaminosis* means a condition resulting from vitamin effects.) It must be noted that the water-soluble vitamins, such as the B complex and Vitamin C, may also cause harmful effects on the body when taken in excessive amounts. Their toxicity, however, is not because of their water solubility alone.

Vitamins and Nutrition

It is difficult to separate vitamins from other elements of nutrition
—the two are intimately related. Nevertheless, we have decided
to limit this book to a discussion of vitamins. The other aspects
of nutrition—such as caloric intake, a balanced diet, proteins,
carbohydrates, and fats—will be discussed briefly in Chapter V
and mentioned in the remainder of this book when necessary for
our discussion of vitamins.

The concept of exact nutrient requirements as expressed in
tables is an illusion. Robert Goodhart (see Primary Sources) has
stated, "Since the quantitative nutrient requirements are dependent upon such things as physical activity, endocrine activity,
efficiency of utilization, rate of growth, composition of the diet
and the like, considerable variation in requirements is to be expected and does in fact exist." Comparable factors are known to
influence vitamin requirements also.

Severe malnutrition is accompanied by vitamin deficiencies,
and both must be treated together. In an extreme case treated by
one of us (Paul Bach-y-Rita), the patient, a five-year-old girl living
in a mountainous region of southern Mexico, looked like a two-
or three-year-old "retarded" child. She could not walk, was virtually unresponsive, scratched herself continuously, and had acute
eye symptoms. The basis of her problem was a severe allergy to
milk. Therefore, she was fed only a corn gruel. Occasionally she

was given some food with a small amount of milk, and each time almost died from diarrhea and other allergic effects. Such cases are extremely difficult to treat, especially as outpatients, but her parents absolutely refused to allow her to be hospitalized. Vitamin therapy and nutritional supplements produced dramatic improvements. She was soon able to walk, her eyes cleared, and she became much more responsive. However, she was occasionally given some food containing milk, and each time she reacted as severely as before. This see-saw battle continued for five months, with the parents continuing to refuse hospitalization. She died during a severe allergic reaction.

It was difficult to separate her vitamin deficiency from the malnutrition, and both were related to her allergy. The doctor often is confronted by a disease state in which the vitamin deficiency is part of the problem and cannot be treated in isolation. However, relatively uncomplicated cases of vitamin deficiency are often found. These can be due to a lack of intake of a sufficient quantity of the vitamins in the body, to environmental factors (e.g., lack of sunlight leading to Vitamin D deficiency), or to the inability of the body to adequately use the vitamins.

As the importance of vitamins became accepted, vitamins began to appear in foods as additives. At the turn of the century, the principal concern of nutritionists was to supply an adequate intake of calories. As vitamins were discovered and their importance appreciated, an effort was made to supply an adequate dietary vitamin intake. However, it became apparent that a standard diet often could not supply sufficient vitamins. For example, in climates with limited sunlight, Vitamin D deficiencies were more likely to occur.

The development of inexpensive methods of manufacturing vitamins made the next logical step possible: to add vitamins to the foods that the potentially vitamin-deficient person was likely to eat. The addition of Vitamin D to milk and infant formulas has practically eliminated Vitamin D deficiencies in many countries. Margarine, white flour, rice, corn and other cereal grains, breakfast foods and beverages are among the foods that are now so enriched.

Not all persons benefit equally from the enrichment program. For example, Goodhart pointed out that the sedentary urban adult who can afford other foods and who does not wish to gain weight consumes comparatively small quantities of cereals and is little affected by the enrichment program. Some of these persons may require supplemental vitamin therapy. Furthermore, since Vitamin D is added to a number of foods, excess of Vitamin D now poses a problem. This will be further discussed in the section on vitamins in Infancy and Childhood (pp. 61 ff.).

Recommended Dietary Allowances (RDA's)

The RDA (see Glossary) for any given nutrient, be it vitamin, mineral, protein, etc., is the result of a complicated government action. Simply stated, the RDA for any given substance is the official government estimate of the amount of essential nutrients each person (infant, child, adult, female, male) in a healthy population needs to consume daily in order to assure proper physiological functioning. By this very definition, one can see that the RDA is no magic number that everyone can agree upon. Indeed, there is much room for argument because of the potential for great variations in requirements in any individual. Thus, the establishment of RDA's should only be considered as a public health guideline, and not as an inviolable nutritional number. In fact, the experts who draft the RDA guidelines every five years recognize that for the essential elements like vitamins they must err on the high side of vitamin requirements to allow for the upper needs of our population.

Another important feature of the RDA's is that they are *recommendations* as to how much of any given nutrient should be present in the foods that are ordinarily consumed. The RDA's are not intended to dictate the amount of each nutrient that should be present in our food. This point is often missed by both the believers and critics of the RDA's. Since RDA's appear to be so widely used and quoted, it may be useful to outline the specific procedures that are followed every five years to arrive at the "new" RDA's.

The primary responsibility for setting up RDA's is that of the prestigious National Academy of Sciences (NAS) through the National Research Council (NRC). A special Food and Nutrition Board of the NAS/NRC then appoints a committee charged with the responsibility of drafting the new RDA's. The committee is composed of experts in nutritional sciences, with usually special expertise in a given area of nutrition. Each specialist (e.g., an expert on Vitamin C) is then asked to review the RDA drafts that already exist and suggest revisions if deemed necessary. This review and revision process may involve special subcommittees. The suggestions are then consolidated and submitted to the main RDA committee for comment. The committee may send its draft out to other experts for further comment if required. When the full RDA committee is satisfied with the resulting draft, the recommendations are passed on to the Food and Nutrition Board for another review. Revisions and comments are again incorporated. A special committee of this board then reviews the documents and finally passes it on to the NAS/NRC for publication as a monograph (which can be obtained from the U.S. Printing Office).

Does such a complicated and extensive process guarantee that the final recommendations are faultless? Of course not, since the very nature of the consensus needed to determine the RDA's eliminates minority reports and dissenting opinions. Most, if not all, of the men and women who work at this thankless task draw upon many pieces of nutritional evidence in arriving at their decisions and recommendations. Animal data as well as human studies go into the deliberations. Even in the best cases information on human needs for vitamins such as E and K are limited. The experts themselves will recognize that estimates of allowances must be based on lowest intake of the substance by any given segment of our population, or must be derived from results on experimental animals. Most of the information contained in the current 1974 issue of RDA's is derived from human studies, but not necessarily from well-controlled scientific experimentation.

A considerable amount of subjective judgment enters into the final RDA figures for many substances. This judgment is widely made for vitamin RDA's.

For example, the RDA for Vitamin C in the seventh edition of the RDA listing was 60 mg for adult males. In the new edition (1973–74) the RDA has been reduced to 45 mg/day for adults. This reduction in RDA was not based on animal studies but upon clinical investigations in man. Based on the amount of Vitamin C needed to prevent scurvy (see Glossary) (probably less than 10 mg/day), and considering the metabolic turnover of the vitamin in the body (30 mg/day would replenish the amount metabolized in healthy individuals), it was concluded that 45 mg/day would be adequate to assure a sufficient pool of the vitamin in healthy men. Yet, even with this reduction in RDA (which surely offends some Vitamin C advocates), the U.S. RDA for this vitamin still is at least 50 percent greater than the standards set by Canada, the United Kingdom, and the World Health Organization!

For many years laissez-faire philosophy governed the manufacture, distribution, promotion, and sale of vitamins in the United States. Whatever government guidelines or restrictions there were, they in no way offered serious limitations on our typical American romance with filling any need that could be found. Consequently, more and more manufacturers entered the field of vitamin production and sales. Increasingly, promotion around the country began to ring of "Indian Snake Oil" claims and tactics. Hence, it was not surprising that as vitamin advertising and consumer patterns began to suggest to our elected and appointed officials that there was consumer fraud being practiced and that Americans might be poisoning themselves with vitamin overdosage, stricter laws and measures were advocated to protect Americans from the hazards of self-medication.

In part, the prominence of vitamin RDA's reflects this concern. But they have hardly eliminated controversy.

For example, the assigned RDA for Vitamin E is 4 to 15 International Units (I.U.) (see Glossary). Some believe the value is too low. Others feel that a true Vitamin E deficiency is a very rare occurrence. Yet others proclaim that no one has any hard scientific evidence proving our needs for Vitamin E, let alone assigning dietary requirements. And finally, there are those who state that Vitamin E should not even carry a vitamin designation.

Is there anything wrong with such a careful and obviously elaborate system for arriving at "Recommended Dietary Allowances?" Probably not, as long as it is agreed what is meant by the "average" person for whom the RDA was designed. Of course, there is no such thing as "an average adult male or female." The "average" American is a statistical construct and bears no necessary correspondence to the individual reading these words. One should be interested in what *one's* body needs, what *one's* body does, and what *one's* extraordinary and unique chemistry requires.

Part of the problem arises from the fact that the RDA is assumed to be needed for the healthy individual to *maintain* his health, that is, to avoid vitamin deficiencies. However, is it not conceivable that when a body is under unusual stress, or is recovering from surgery, or is subjected to certain noxious substances, the RDA may have to be increased (or decreased)?

Professor Roger Williams of the Clayton Institute of the University of Texas has spent a lifetime investigating the question of biochemical individuality and nutritional needs. He presents evidence from animal studies that Vitamin C requirements of guinea pigs may vary twentyfold. Cannot such a variation also exist in man? However, it is presently impractical to routinely and precisely define subtle or unique individual differences and variations in body chemistry as it relates to specific vitamin status.

Environmental stresses take many forms. Modern urban man probably will live with air pollution for a long time. Air pollutants may include oxidants, and these oxidants, through their hyperoxygen effect on tissues, may produce serious lung damage. What does all this have to do with RDA's? There is some evidence showing that high doses of Vitamin E, through its antioxidant (see Glossary) effect, can protect against lung and tissue damage associated with oxidizing pollutants and ozone. Who then will tell us what constitutes the RDA for a man who lives in such a potentially toxic environment?

The RDA's for vitamins are important guidelines for all of us. However, they are not intended as absolute nutritional dictates.

II

EXAMINING SOME COMMON BELIEFS

Vitamin C and
the Common Cold

When Vitamin C (ascorbic acid) is discussed in most academic, research, and lay circles, it is invariably in relation to its use (or abuse) in the prevention or treatment of the common cold. The publication (1970) of a book by Nobel Laureate Linus Pauling (see Primary Sources) dealing with the subject undoubtedly has been the stimulus for a resurgence of interest in this controversial medical and nutritional question. This is not to say that the use of Vitamin C in colds had not been looked at before. As early as 1942, the use of ascorbic acid in preventing or treating the common cold was investigated. Most of the studies that characterized the period from 1942 to 1971 were not well designed or controlled studies. ("Controlled" refers to the use of inactive placebos [see Glossary], as well as the substance under test, on groups of patients. Neither the subject nor the investigator knows which substance is being given—until the study has been completed. This is a so-called double blind study [see Glossary].)

However, the modern era of research on the use of ascorbic acid in preventing and treating colds really began in the early 1970's. What have been the results of these up-to-date, carefully controlled studies? In one trial involving 818 volunteers, 1 to 4 grams of ascorbic acid daily did not significantly reduce the frequency of colds compared to the results in the placebo group. However, the total number of disability days ("confined to the house") was higher in the placebo group, indicating some beneficial effects of ascorbic acid as measured by this parameter. However, a later study by the same investigators, involving a final number of 1,171 subjects, failed to show a beneficial effect from the use of 0.25 to 8 grams of the vitamin, either in the number or severity of the illnesses. Another trial using 3 grams per day also failed to protect volunteers against a flu virus. Similar failures of Vitamin C were noted in clinical trials involving children. In one of these studies the frequency of toxic colds (sore throat, headache, fever, malaise) was actually increased in girls taking the 0.5 gram dose of the chemical. The *severity* of head colds was reduced (in girls only) with 0.2 grams of the vitamin, but the *duration* of variety-symptom colds was longer when the dose was 0.5 grams.

Obviously, the difficulty in assessing the "severity," "duration," or episodes of illness makes quantification of such studies difficult. But when these modern studies were reviewed by *The Medical Letter* (October 11, 1974), the conclusion was "that large doses of Vitamin C do not prevent colds, and evidence suggesting the vitamin might reduce the severity or duration of colds is not convincing."

The head of a large New York Medical Center recently reviewed the clinical reports dealing with the pros and cons of Vitamin C therapy for the common cold. His survey covered material published during the period from 1942 to 1974. He reached the following conclusions: (1) The vitamin is virtually ineffective as a cold-preventer or cold-shortener. (2) When the vitamin does reduce the severity of symptoms, the effects are quantitatively too small to warrant long-term consumption of the chemical. At the best, the survey of twelve studies by eleven different centers revealed that cold symptoms and malaise were reduced by the amount of sixth-tenths of a day per year on the average. Since long-term toxicity (see Glossary) offers potential dangers (see below), one wonders whether such marginal clinical effects are worth the risk.

Similar conclusions were reached by another group of investigators following study of 311 government employees. If there is a decrease in severity of cold symptoms, "it is clinically insignificant." This conclusion was based on their clinical studies where subjects received 3 grams of ascorbic acid per day (or, when they caught a cold, 6 grams per day). Of course, the same attitude can be taken toward the use of common cold remedies containing aspirin, antihistamines (see Glossary), decongestants, etc., which can also cause adverse reactions, although these drugs may alleviate the symptoms of the colds.

Drs. Michael Dykes and Paul Meier also have made a careful and critical review of the published scientific literature dealing with ascorbic acid and the common cold (see Primary Sources). They reviewed the clinical literature published between 1938 and March 1975. Their review must certainly be read by the serious reader who wishes to get another critical view of this medical controversy. In brief, they concluded that there is no clear, reproducible pattern of efficacy of Vitamin C in preventing or treating the common cold. We particularly agree with their conclusion that "until such time as pharmacologic doses of ascorbic acid have been shown to have obvious, important clinical value in the prevention and treatment of the common cold, and to be safe in a large varied population, we cannot advocate its unrestricted use for such purposes."

In contrast to this conclusion, Dr. C. W. M. Wilson of Dublin Trinity College believes there is adequate reason to recommend supplemental ascorbic acid therapy in treating the common cold. His analysis of nine controlled clinical studies (including his own) prompts him to the opposite conclusion made by other reviewers examining the same studies (see Primary Sources). Why such a major discrepancy when scientists are asked to appraise the same set of published data? This enigma plagues the research (or lack of it) relating to the Vitamin C–common cold debate. Partisanship may play a role, despite the professed objectivity of the reviewers. We have reviewed not only the majority of the original studies under debate but also the independent reviews and assessments of these papers by competent scientists. Our view is that it would be a great mistake for the layman to risk the real hazards of ascorbic acid toxicity in exchange for the very questionable minor benefits, if any, of reduction of severity of cold symptoms.

There are many additional questions that arise from the Vitamin C–common cold dilemma. Dr. T. W. Anderson of Toronto (see Primary Sources), who has studied the problem extensively, has reported that part of the difficulty of studying the responses to Vitamin C is that there are different tissue saturation levels of the vitamin when studies are begun.

The relationship between the amount of Vitamin C consumed and blood levels is critical. Apparently it is difficult to raise blood levels of the vitamin above 1.39 mg per 100 ml of blood. This maximum blood level can be reached with small doses of 90 to 100 mg per day taken over seven to eight weeks. Under stress or infection, saturation may occur at a higher level. This will vary from individual to individual; hence there would be varying effects produced by any given dose. Everyone agrees that man (as well as the gorilla and other species) cannot synthesize Vitamin C. However, the vitamin must be replenished continuously in order to maintain "normal" tissue levels. In certain conditions (e.g., following surgery or infections) there is a demonstrated depletion of these cellular stores of Vitamin C, and increased consumption is required to restore desired levels. Is the common cold one of these conditions?

One rationale for the use of large doses of Vitamin C is that the chemical produces a fleeting or transient effect before it is excreted; and there is no need to assume that any absolute tissue or blood levels of the chemical are required. (The total body pool of ascorbic acid is approximately 1,500 mg. As little as 10 mg/day given by mouth is sufficient to prevent or cure scurvy in individuals who were totally deprived of the vitamin for periods from 84 to 97 days—a procedure that experimentally induces the symptoms of scurvy.)

The advocates of the use of ascorbic acid for the prevention and treatment of the common cold also emphasize that there is normally a strong positive correlation between plasma and white cell content of the vitamin. During a cold, this relationship changes (i.e., there is less Vitamin C in the white cells). Doses of 500 to 2,000 mg of Vitamin C raise the white cell ascorbic acid level in young females following recovery from colds. During the peak symptoms of the cold, only the highest dose can produce "normal" levels of the vitamin in white blood cells and blood. In males, a still higher dose may be needed to maintain normal white cell concentrations of the vitamin. Apparently, an inverse relationship exists between the severity of cold symptoms and the ascorbic acid content of the white cells, at least in colds characterized by respiratory tract inflammation. Yet, the specific clinical protective role of the vitamin is not that dramatic as revealed by carefully controlled studies mentioned earlier.

Thus, while we have precise knowledge of the amount of vitamin in the body, of how much is needed to maintain stores, of what levels are associated with scurvy, of the metabolic pathways for elimination (and much more), application of these facts to the common cold is hazardous. How massive doses of Vitamin C act to allegedly fight colds is unknown. The consensus is that if it does have an effect, it is not acting as a vitamin but as a chemical with druglike properties. (The presence of "druglike properties" may discourage the use of massive doses of ascorbic acid by people who are generally not prone to take "drugs" regardless of their disguise or origin!) For example, in high doses ascorbic acid has a weak antihistamine effect. Thus, the runny noses and upper respiratory tract symptoms that may be decreased by massive doses of the vitamin may be due to a classical antihistamine-like action!

If one assumes, for the sake of argument, that the recommended massive doses of ascorbic acid are beneficial in treating the common cold, what are the "risks" associated with such therapy? The reported side effects are numerous; most may be dismissed as minor or of rare occurrence. Some are substantial and warrant exposure. These effects may be especially important for the chronic user of high doses of the vitamin.

(1) *Anemia.* High doses of Vitamin C have been reported to inactivate Vitamin B_{12}. This is discussed in the section on Vitamins in Relation to Other Substances (pp. 85 ff.). Vitamin B_{12} is

necessary for normal blood cell function. Its absence can lead to certain anemias.

(2) *Stones.* One of the metabolic by-products of ascorbic acid is dehydroascorbic acid, and its end product oxalate (see Glossary). Increased consumption of ascorbic acid can raise the blood levels of oxalate, and this may cause the formation of oxalate stones in the kidneys and bladder. Also, taking large amounts of ascorbic acid results in a more acid urine and this may cause precipitation of urate or cystine stones in the urinary tract. This may occur more frequently in individuals who are predisposed to such stone formation (gout).

(3) *Blood clotting.* High doses of ascorbic acid may interact with certain anticoagulant drugs such as warfarin (Coumadin) to reduce the desired effect of the latter substance (which is to prolong bleeding time, thus reducing the chance of clot formation). If one is taking warfarin or similar drugs (given by prescription), it would not be wise to take high doses of ascorbic acid without the specific approval of a physician.

(4) *Mucolytic action.* Other evidence suggests that high doses of ascorbic acid can cause a mucolytic (i.e., destruction of mucous lining or membranes) effect which can affect the thickness of the cervical mucous lining. This change may in turn affect fertilization mechanisms.

(5) Vitamin C can interact with many other drugs. (See section on Vitamins in Relation to Other Substances.)

(6) *Diarrhea.* Consumption of 1 gram of ascorbic acid per day may produce diarrhea. Abdominal pain (colic) has also been reported.

In conclusion, the burden of proof continues to be on the advocates of the use of these megadoses of Vitamin C. No compelling scientific evidence is available to justify the use of such a marginally effective (if at all) agent which, in susceptible individuals, may cause adverse reactions. It is also worth noting that Linus Pauling, in his own book, declares: "I do not know how effective this regimen really is." Despite the research effort being devoted to the problem, the layman should be cautioned on the use of megadoses of Vitamin C to treat the common cold.

Vitamin E and the Heart

In all probability the advocacy and use of large doses of alpha-tocopherol (see Glossary) (Vitamin E) in disorders of cardiovascular function is based not on the agent's vitamin properties but upon its pharmacological actions.

Over a period of almost two decades, a multitude of human studies have purported to show the effectiveness of alpha-tocopherol in the treatment of angina pectoris, myocardial infarction, congestive heart failure, Buerger's disease (thromboangitis obliterans), acute thrombophlebitis, intermittent claudication, varicose veins, and other peripheral vascular diseases.

Despite such widespread clinical observations, the use of alpha-tocopherol in cardiovascular disorders still appears to be based on hope and speculation rather than a firm biochemical or physiological reason.

This section will focus on a survey of recent studies dealing with the use of alpha-tocopherol, based upon specific actions on metabolic and physiological functions of the heart and blood vessels.

One of the alleged therapeutic applications of alpha-tocopherol is in the treatment of peripheral vascular disorders characterized by insufficient blood flow to extremities. However, these actions are not readily demonstrated in controlled clinical studies.

There is a tendency to ascribe the variety of vascular effects of alpha-tocopherol to its antioxidant properties, its role in the synthesis of coenzyme A (see Glossary) and of ATP, and its role in the maintenance of cellular succinate oxidation. Unfortunately, these claims are not readily apparent from clinical studies.

The ideal peripheral vasodilator (see Glossary) does not exist for the treatment of peripheral vascular disorders. The spectrum of vascular actions of alpha-tocopherol is not that prominent or predictable, and therefore has not been widely exploited nor accepted. Certainly, it should not be taken for such conditions without a physician's supervision.

Modern controlled clinical trials have failed to demonstrate a protective or beneficial action of alpha-tocopherol in angina pectoris and coronary artery disease. These and other studies were recently reviewed by Professor Robert E. Olson of St. Louis University School of Medicine (see Primary Sources). He concluded that there is no compelling scientific evidence to suggest the use of high doses of Vitamin E in various cardiac disorders.

It is now known that increased dietary use of polyunsaturated fats (as advocated by the American Heart Association) increases the need for Vitamin E and therefore may result in the inability to achieve adequate blood levels of alpha-tocopherol. In addition, the fatty acids released by polyunsaturates are extremely vulnerable to peroxidation (see Glossary). The presence of alpha-tocopherol prevents this oxidation. But in the process there is a degradation of the antioxidant. Therefore, this interaction between alpha-tocopherol and polyunsaturates must be appreciated in planning dietary regimens for cardiovascular patients.

Concern exists over the possible interaction of alpha-tocopherol and digitalis glycosides. Until this controversy is resolved, it is suggested that patients receiving digitalis be carefully dosed with alpha-tocopherol. A reduction of the glycoside (see Glossary) dose may be required.

The possibility of interaction of alpha-tocopherol with other agents used in the treatment of cardiovascular disease also must be considered by the attending physician.

Vitamin E and Blood Disorders

While there is no compelling scientific evidence implicating Vitamin E deficiency as a cause of sterility, heart disease, hypertension (see Glossary), atherosclerosis (see Glossary), or a host of other diseases, there are certain rare blood conditions that have been associated with Vitamin E deficiency. These include: megaloblastic anemia (see Glossary) in children, hemolytic anemia (see Glossary) in premature infants, red blood cell fragility (associated with a genetic lack of beta lipoproteins [see Glossary]). An apparently clear deficiency state has been defined in infants fed on infant formulas. These conditions respond well to the recommended daily amount of Vitamin E. As little as 2 to 10 I.U. of the vitamin may prevent the destruction of red blood cells in susceptible children. The damage to red blood cells caused by excessive oxygen tension (presumably due to formation of tissue peroxides) has also been shown to be prevented by Vitamin E (and other antioxidants). However, unless one is exposed to an artificially high oxygen atmosphere (as was used in the early Mercury Astronaut Project), there is little likelihood that such damage to red cells occurs.

Vitamin E, Human Fertility, and Sexuality

A persistent myth among laymen is that Vitamin E possesses some magical quality that restores or maintains human sexual function, or is necessary in maintaining fertility (or preventing sterility). It must be stated firmly and unequivocally that Vitamin E is not needed to maintain fertility or sexual function in either male or female. Neither does this substance have the ability to cure or reverse human infertility. Even the most enthusiastic supporter of the miracles that Vitamin E is alleged to bring about cannot point to one shred of evidence in man that Vitamin E functions as a fertility factor or has some property for maintaining or enhancing human sexual performance or potency. This often-perpetuated myth has been universally and repeatedly condemned and refuted by every responsible reviewer of the scientific facts.

Despite these disclaimers and evidence, the laymen still picture Vitamin E as the fertility vitamin. Why? The origins of Vitamin E discovery provide the answer.

Vitamin E was discovered in 1922 by Evans and Bishop. They noted that a specific fat-soluble factor (later identified as alpha-tocopherol) was necessary in the diet of rats if they were to reproduce normally. Thus, male rats deliberately deprived of Vitamin E become sterile. (Reproductive disorders also may occur in mice and guinea pigs deprived of Vitamin E.) In fact, because the substance they identified was critical to reproduction in rats, they gave it the name tocopherol (see Glossary), which is derived from the Greek words *tokos*, meaning childbirth, and *phero* meaning to bring. These classical and elegant experiments on rats, while valid and reproducible, do not apply to human biology, or to many other mammalian species. Vitamin E has been tried in the treatment of human infertility with negative results. It has been tried as an agent to prevent spontaneous abortions in women and has failed. The myth of Vitamin E as a fertility vitamin in humans should be buried once and for all.

Vitamin D— Necessary but to Be Used with Caution

Vitamin D is important to human nutrition because it is involved as a regulator of the absorption, metabolism (see Glossary), and utilization of the essential minerals, calcium and phosphate. Since all cells require calcium for proper functioning, the action of Vitamin D is widespread and critical to good health. In fact, Vitamin D is now considered by some scientists to be a hormone (see Glossary). Recent studies have shown that the active Vitamin D metabolite has a mode of action similar to the classical steroid hormones (see Glossary). The recognition that the kidney is obligatory, as an endocrine organ, for the elaboration of the active metabolite, opens up the possibility of developing therapeutic measures for bone abnormalities associated with chronic kidney failure. These diseases may involve a defect in the production of the kidney hormone. Furthermore, a reinvestigation of other diseases, such as Vitamin-D–resistant rickets, is called for.

The main disease that results from a Vitamin D deficiency, rickets (see Glossary), is an extremely rare event in the United States. The U.S. Department of Health, Education and Welfare conducted a survey between 1968 and 1970 of the prevalence of Vitamin D deficiency of low-income groups (a segment of our population always suspected of having nutritional deficiencies). The survey found that there was an insignificant number of children with clinical manifestation of Vitamin D deficiency (namely, rickets). This surprising finding probably is best explained by the fact that as the result of the widespread use of Vitamin D in milk and infant formulas, Vitamin D deficiency is unlikely to occur, except in the rarest instances of gross nutritional neglect or hereditary disorders.

It is possible, however, that true Vitamin D deficiency can result from nondietary factors, namely, lack of exposure to ultraviolet rays necessary for the conversion of the chemical precursors of Vitamin D that occur in the skin. This relative deficiency has been reported for individuals who work and live in offices and homes that largely have fluorescent lighting, and therefore are deprived of the necessary ultraviolet radiation. During the appearance of heavy industrial smog in England and northern Europe, Vitamin D deficiency rickets was reported to be increased because there was a filtering out of the necessary ultraviolet rays by the air pollutants.

Another important group of individuals may develop signs and symptoms of Vitamin D deficiency due to hereditary conditions that result in low phosphate levels in the blood (phosphates are linked to calcium metabolism), or who suffer from kidney disease resulting in urinary loss of phosphate, or other dysfunctions (see Glossary). These are rare conditions, and a physician must be consulted to determine whether or not the clinical signs of Vitamin D deficiency are due to true lack of the vitamin or due to the rare hereditary defects in calcium or phosphate metabolism.

If rickets, due to a dietary deficiency of Vitamin D, is so rare, and there is no other proven indication* for the use of the vita-

---

*The use of Vitamin D in patients who have calcium deficiencies resulting from malfunctioning livers associated with alcoholism has been reported as an application of Vitamin D in a non-rickets situation. These large doses of the vitamin are only useful in such specific liver diseases that affect normal Vitamin D metabolism. Such high doses in people who do not suffer specific liver diseases can cause harmful effects.

min in man, why take supplementary Vitamin D?

No responsible authority or agency involved with public health and nutrition advocates the use of Vitamin D above the amount needed to prevent Vitamin D dependent rickets. The RDA for Vitamin D is 400 I.U. (10 micrograms [see Glossary]). It should be emphasized that as little as 100 I.U. per day can prevent rickets, but better mineralization of the bone in infants occurs with the higher amount. Also, the amount required for older children and adults may be decreased with sufficient exposure to sunlight. The position of the National Academy of Sciences is that normal healthy adults meet their requirements of Vitamin D by nondietary sources, and therefore no dietary or supplementary recommendation is necessary.

Since it is clearly established that we are not suffering the ravages of Vitamin D deficiency, is there any reason for, or danger in, taking higher amounts of Vitamin D "just to be on the safe side"? The consensus of responsible authorities, including the National Academy of Sciences, is that there is no reason for taking supplemental or excessive amounts of Vitamin D. It is also agreed that excessive amounts of this substance are dangerous to infants, children, and adults alike, and should be avoided.

Excess amounts of Vitamin D (e.g., 2,000 I.U./day) for prolonged periods has been well documented to produce severe side effects in infants and adults. These adverse reactions are detailed in another section of this book (pp. 96 ff.).

The important thing for the reader to understand and appreciate is that ingestion of Vitamin D in excess of the recommended amounts (probably 100 to 400 I.U.) provides no extra benefit to the body, and in fact larger excesses may be demonstrably harmful and dangerous. Some exciting and new research on Vitamin D and its metabolites is being conducted. However, the precise mode and mechanism of action of these substances is still not fully understood. While these new findings will enhance our knowledge about this vitamin, we must appreciate the facts that are already established, including what is needed to prevent rickets and what happens when we take an excessive amount.

Vitamin D and Heart Attack

Most of the toxicity that occurs with excessive vitamin consumption has been described and is generally well known by physicians and nutritionists, and hopefully by an increasing number of consumers. However, there remains an area of controversy that requires exploration. This relates to the question of whether or not Vitamin D consumption may be linked to heart attack, or, more precisely, myocardial infarction (see Glossary).

For several years, investigators have been studying the possible link between Vitamin A and D consumption, cholesterol (see Glossary) metabolism and the incidence of heart disease in man. Until now, no definitive study has been made to permit any conclusions. However, a recent report by Linden (see Primary Sources) now suggests that long-term consumption of Vitamin D, of the order of 30 micrograms (or 1200 I.U.) per day, may be a precipitating factor or cause of myocardial infarction. This conclusion was based upon investigation of medical records drawn from the Central Bureau of Statistics from Northern Norway.

The results of this analysis indicated that those patients who had suffered heart attacks had a higher average daily consumption of Vitamin D than all other groups. The differences in vitamin intake per day for males and females who suffered heart attacks was statistically higher than corresponding matched controls who had not suffered cardiac disorders.

The authors of this study point out that a critical level of Vitamin D might be involved, and they recommend that efforts be made to restrict the intake of Vitamin D except from its production by the skin through the action of sunlight. They advocate that the concept of Vitamin D preparations as tonics should be dispelled, and careful consideration be given to restricting the ease of acquiring such preparations through commercial sale. This is a thought-provoking report that will undoubtedly influence attitudes toward the promiscuous use of Vitamin D, either to fortify foods or in commercial vitamin preparations.

Natural versus Synthetic Vitamins

One has only to scan the advertisements in health food magazines to appreciate the attempts to convince the vitamin-consuming public that natural vitamins are better than their synthetic counterparts.

Generally, "natural" vitamins refer to vitamins as they exist in nature. Thus, the Vitamin C in "rose hips" is alleged to have different properties and effects than the equivalent amount of synthetic ascorbic acid. The Vitamin E present in wheat germ oil is thought to exert different effects than the equivalent amount of synthetic alpha-tocopherol. The Vitamin A in carrot juice is held to be superior to the chemical entity derived synthetically.

Is there any scientific proof that there indeed exists a difference between natural and synthetic vitamins?

Chemically, Vitamin C is ascorbic acid which consists of six carbon atoms, eight hydrogens and six oxygens ($C_6H_8O_6$) arranged in a molecular configuration unique to this substance. This molecular figure print can be confirmed by a variety of chemical and physical measurements. The chemist starts with known chemical entities en route to synthesizing ascorbic acid. The purity and identity of his efforts can be checked and confirmed by precise methods which can detect contamination, impurities, or instability. Exact qualities that must be met to satisfy the label "Vitamin C," or ascorbic acid, for use in humans, are defined by the United States Pharmacopoeia Commission. Such tested and certified ascorbic acid may be labeled "Vitamin C, U.S.P." Ascorbic acid not meeting these rigid requirements of purity cannot be labeled "U.S.P.," although one can buy non-U.S.P. ascorbic acid from chemical supply companies.

If synthetic Vitamin C is so precisely characterized chemically, why do health food advocates claim that Vitamin C found in nature is "different"? If in fact it were different, it could not be called Vitamin C. What is being claimed and promoted is that the actions of synthetic Vitamin C are not the same as those obtained with the natural (and usually more expensive!) forms of the vitamin. There is no scientific evidence to support such a belief. One hundred milligrams of synthetic ascorbic acid U.S.P. has the same biochemical and physiological action of 100 mg of Vitamin C obtained from "rose hips" (which are derived from the dried bulb portion of a rose following blossoming).

It must be emphasized that natural rose hips are not pure Vitamin C. Rose hip preparations may contain only about 2 percent by weight of the pure vitamin. Moreover, many commercial preparations contain added synthetic Vitamin C. In fact, if they were not "spiked" with this synthetic Vitamin C, the rose hip tablet might have to be extraordinarily large in size to contain the desired amount of ascorbic acid. Bulk rose hips, as supplied to health-food-store processers, are often labeled as containing only 50 percent ascorbic acid. Yet, when the consumer buys the preparation, the label usually is misleading since it reads "Rose Hips Vitamin C." Interestingly, present federal and local laws do not require a percentage breakdown of the rose hips versus pure ascorbic acid content of the rose hip tablet to be placed on the label. Another misleading aspect of rose hips is that a 500-mg rose hip tablet, for example, may be advertised as containing 1050 percent of the adult RDA Vitamin-C requirement. Yet on a milligram basis, approximately 475 mg of pure ascorbic acid provides the same percentage of the RDA. Examination of the natural-B-vitamins preparations reveals the same misleading information. The commercial procedure of loading the yeast or other natural-B source with synthetic B vitamins is often done with no indication on the label.

In popular health food magazines, much is made of the alleged difference in chromatographic appearance of synthetic and natural Vitamin C. (A chromatogram is a color "fingerprint" of a substance obtained by visualization of the substance by specially treated paper.) The pictures of such chromatograms indicate the synthetic Vitamin C is uniform and symmetrical in appearance. The vitamin derived from "natural sources" has more irregular surfaces and edges. This difference is always interpreted in favor of the "natural" vitamin, i.e., it "looks alive," etc. What is never mentioned is the fact that such irregularities suggest chemical impurity or presence of other substances which result in a pattern more complex than the pure synthetic material. Thus, natural Vitamin C is thought to have different properties in the body owing to these additional co-factors. No controlled scientific studies exist to suggest that such co-factors (if indeed they do exist) allow the vitamin to exert any different effect on cell processes than that obtained by the pure single chemical entity, ascorbic acid.

These observations are not to discount the possibility that differences cannot exist between Vitamin C preparations, even if derived from totally synthetic sources. For many years, pharmacologists and physiologists argued that ingestion of 100 mg of any chemically pure substance should predictably result in equal absorption, distribution, effect, and metabolism. This concept of "generic equivalency" recently has been under intense scrutiny, however. What is being shown in man is that ingestion of various brands of 5-grain aspirin U.S.P., or 0.25 mg digitalis U.S.P., or 250 mg tetracycline U.S.P., for example, does not mean each brand will be equally effective. Thus, all "5-grain aspirin, U.S.P." contain the same amount of acetylsalicylic acid (aspirin). To be so labeled, exact standards must be met; yet all brands of such aspirin are not necessarily therapeutically equal in action. The reason is that some 5-grain U.S.P. aspirin are compounded and

formulated differently than others. The differences in tablet making (inert materials, such as lactose, compression factors, etc.)
can vary tremendously from the cheapest brand of aspirin U.S.P.
to the brands with high quality control. This applies to many
drugs and substances, including vitamins, even though carrying
identical labels of content.

The subtle or marked differences in these manufacturing formulation processes can often result in great variability in therapeutic effect due to poorer or better absorption, lower or higher
blood and tissue levels, etc. As the result of such modern research (called pharmacokinetics [see Glossary]), we know that all
generically equivalent substances are not therapeutically equivalent. The differences between generically equivalent agents usually resolve down to questions of bioavailability (see Glossary).
(This term refers to the actual biological availability to the cells
of the body of the substance after it is taken.)

In this context, a tablet containing 100 mg of a vitamin may not
necessarily produce its desired action on the body if it does not
properly disintegrate, dissolve, be transported into the blood,
and reach the desired therapeutic blood level. A properly formulated tablet containing 100 mg of the identical substance, because it does disintegrate, dissolve, is transported, and reaches
a desired blood level, will produce the desired or anticipated
biological action.

The federal government and many consumer groups have advocated generic (chemical) equivalency, arguing that chemicals,
drugs, and substances of identical content should not differ in
their actions. (This argument is usually made in the economic
context, since many so-called generic substances are often
cheaper than identically labeled brand-name equivalents.) What
modern research has revealed, however, is that biological or
therapeutic equivalency is what is important. The government
has begun to acknowledge that legally and correctly labeled generic products often result in either inadequate or unpredictable
blood levels and effects, compared to other more extensively
quality-controlled preparations.

While this generic versus therapeutic equivalency debate has focused largely on drugs, it is now clear that the scientific arguments developed also are applicable to vitamins.

Thus, purchase of a cheap generic Vitamin C tablet labeled "100 mg Vitamin C" does not guarantee that the user will get the equivalent biological effect as that obtainable with a more highly quality-controlled (and thus possibly more expensive) "100 mg Vitamin C" tablet manufactured and sold under a brand name. If the preparations are equally stable in tablet form, dissolve equally at stomach acidity, are absorbed equally, equal blood and tissue levels are obtained, and equal therapeutic (e.g., anti-scurvy) actions are achieved, then the two preparations are "therapeutically equivalent." It obviously would be best to buy the cheaper of the two such therapeutically equivalent vitamin preparations. However, the consumer usually does not know how the various vitamin preparations rank in this regard and is usually guided by the promotional skills of the manufacturers and vendor, or by economic considerations. However, in the very near future we may expect that the same research that led to the demise of "generic equivalency" will be applied to vitamins. At this time, there certainly is no proof to indicate the superiority or advantages of "natural vitamins" over that of synthetic vitamins, in terms of biological effects.

The advocates of the superiority of "natural" versus "synthetic" like to cite the chemical fact that in nature, Vitamin E exists as *d*-alpha-tocopherol. The *dl*-form of the vitamin is that usually identified with the chemically synthesized vitamin. (The *d* refers to dextro rotary, i.e., polarized light is deflected to the right when passed through the substance; *dl* means that both dextro and levo (left deflecting) isomers (see Glossary) are present, so-called racemic (see Glossary) mixture.) It has been shown that the *d*-alpha form is 20 to 30 percent higher in biological activity than the racemic form. What the proponents of these facts forget to mention is that *synthetic d*-alpha-tocopherol is also available. There is no difference in the biological activity of the *d*-alpha form found in "nature" and that produced by "synthetic" manipulations. In fact, many derivatives of alpha-tocopherol have been made by the chemist, and these have been studied for their biological activity. Moreover, the "natural"-vitamin advocates usually forget to mention the fact that there are eight naturally occurring forms of Vitamin E. One is the alpha form; the others are given the Greek letters beta, gamma, and delta. All the forms have been found in foods and fats. One rare form is found only in palm oil. Perhaps this will cause a wave of research on the therapeutic use of palm oil!

These considerations do not argue against the validity of obtaining one's vitamins through naturally occurring food sources. If one is able to obtain the minimum Recommended Dietary Allowance of any vitamin through a proper, well-balanced diet, this is the best and "natural" way. If vitamin supplements are prescribed or needed above those obtainable from normal nutritional sources, then one can use synthetic vitamin supplements. Remember, there is no scientific basis to expect any special or miraculous benefits from so-called natural vitamins. They are usually more expensive anyway.

Orthomolecular Medicine and Megavitamin Therapy

Orthomolecular medicine and megavitamin therapy are far from being ordinary household phrases like the Salk vaccine. While these terms are used in some limited circles of the health sciences, they are not understood by most professionals, let alone by the layman to whom such therapy or medicine is being delivered. It is the purpose of this chapter to discuss some of the implications of these two controversial subjects as they apply to the prevention and treatment of disease and the maintenance of good health. We do this because both orthomolecular medicine and megavitamin therapy make extensive use of vitamins in a most unusual way.

The phrases orthomolecular medicine and megavitamin therapy often are used interchangeably. Megavitamin (*mega* = large or great) therapy basically involves the use of vitamins in amounts substantially higher than those stated in the Recommended Dietary Allowances (RDA's) published by the National Academy of Sciences. The phrase "orthomolecular medicine" was coined by Dr. Linus Pauling. His concept is that the treatment of certain diseases may be accomplished by changing the amounts of key substances in the body that are normally present and which are required for the preservation of good health. (*Ortho* = straight, right, or correct; *molecular* = pertaining to chemical structure of substances.)

Megavitamin therapy, while not a new concept in medicine and therapeutics, has received its greatest impetus during the past few years. This has been due in large part to notable individuals (patients and investigators alike) who have advocated the use of large-dose vitamin therapy in the treatment of mental illness, particularly schizophrenia. The treatment for these latter disease states is often referred to as orthomolecular psychiatry. (There is a specialized *Journal of Orthomolecular Psychiatry;* a book by Drs. David Hawkins and Linus Pauling called *Orthomolecular Psychiatry* was published in 1973 [see Primary Sources].)

What is the logic or rationale for the use of massive amounts of vitamins in the treatment of mental illness? Two Canadian psychiatrists, Abram Hoffer and Humphrey Osmond, probably popularized the use of megavitamin therapy as the result of publishing papers on their apparent success in treating schizophrenia with large doses (3 grams) of nicotinic acid. Considerable biochemical rationalization of their treatment was developed. That is, they *hypothesized* that there were defects in the metabolism of certain substances that cause the mental symptoms of schizophrenia. Administering large doses of niacin (a vitamin) are thought to provide a chemical antidote for these toxic substances. Their idea was further supported by the occasional observation that in pellagra (a primary disease resulting from lack of niacin) there may be signs and symptoms resembling those seen in schizophrenia. These concepts and suggested therapy did not fall upon many receptive ears until Dr. Pauling published his famous paper on orthomolecular psychiatry in 1968. The world-famous chemist defined orthomolecular psychiatric therapy as "the treatment of mental disease by provision of optimum molecular environment for the mind." Properly, he noted that the normal functioning of the brain requires the presence and activity of molecules of many different substances. (No one familiar with the physiology of brain function can deny such a broad concept.) What is at issue is his thought that in certain mental disease there may be a deficiency in the brain of such vitamins as thiamin (Vitamin B_1), nicotinic acid (B_3), pyridoxine (B_6), cyanocobalamin (B_{12}), ascorbic acid (Vitamin C), biotin, and folic acid. Moreover, the concept may be equally applied to diseases of the heart, kidney, liver, gut, and other organs.

It would be difficult in a book such as this to review all the appropriate scientific papers that provide evidence pro and con concerning the question of whether or not there is a demonstrated abnormality in vitamin content or function in certain diseases such as mental illness. If there is a need, is the disease satisfactorily treated with the megadoses of the vitamins that Dr. Pauling and his associates advocate?

The question of being able to show conclusively that there is some abnormal deficiency or requirement for certain vitamins (or other key substances) in mental illness is under intense debate and investigation. At this writing, we are unable to discern any compelling, carefully controlled scientific studies that provide convincing evidence that mental illness, particularly schizophrenia, is due to a primary defect in vitamin content, utilization, or metabolism by the brain. Here it should also be noted that most mental illnesses, including schizophrenia, are not caused by a single factor or abnormality. They tend to be complex, mosaic diseases. Thus, even the alleged clinical success (almost all of them anecdotal in description) involving megavitamin therapy, in no way can be extended to all patients suffering the same disease syndrome. This might be analogous to penicillin therapy: it is beneficial in certain infections that are susceptible to the known actions of the antibiotic; yet there are other infections where this known effective drug will not work at all.

However, with penicillin, when it does its job, its use and mechanism are based upon sound, widely recognized, scientifically substantiated observations. With megavitamin therapy, which makes up an important feature of orthomolecular psychiatry, there is no such scientific consensus. Medicine and science do not necessarily advance as the result of scientific consensus. The history of medicine and science are filled with examples where new ideas or treatments were rejected by the existing science establishment at the time of their introduction. Only through persistent, scientifically convincing, reproducible investigations from both the originators of the new concepts and independent observers from other laboratories do these new controversial ideas gain acceptance and universality. Only by such rigorous process of critical examination are the ideas and facts of science hardened and annealed into truths. Thus, many concepts that were widely accepted by authorities as being true and immutable may turn out to be in error, and then they are rejected and dispelled from the body of science. On the other hand, views that are rejected today may, with the application of newer methods of analysis and measurement, emerge as truths. While these processes evolve, caution must be used in accepting emotional pleas, partisan advocacy or criticism, or unsubstantiated or cleverly contrived rationalizations disguising hypothesis and opinion. Hypotheses may be tested and examined. Results that are consistent with the idea may be used to further test the original idea or expand upon it. Conversely, if the results of the examination fail to provide support for the hypothesis, then it must be rejected, or a new question restated and examined again with new approaches. (Unfortunately this formalized method of science is glaringly absent in many of the questions and issues dealt with in this chapter.)

A case in point: In 1973 a special task force of the American Psychiatric Association was asked to study the use of megavitamin therapy in psychiatry. They concluded that "the results and claims of the advocates of megavitamin therapy have not been confirmed by several groups of psychiatrists and psychologists experienced in psychopharmacological research." The task force also pointed out the refusal over the past ten years of proponents of megavitamin therapy to perform scientifically controlled experiments and to have the results reviewed by their peers. The association thus has gone on record to condemn this method of medical management of mental illness.

Such "establishment" criticism and condemnation does not deter the advocates of orthomolecular psychiatry. It is worth noting the following comments from H. N. Ross (see Primary

Sources): "Too many physicians have attempted to use megavitamins by giving inadequate doses of a few vitamins to the wrong people for an insufficient amount of time only to achieve the failure that could be predicted. The use of vitamins in the treatment of psychiatric conditions is only part of the orthomolecular treatment and takes knowledge, skill, and experience."

Such explanations for the failure of an advocated therapy are not new or confined to megavitamin therapy. They may be valid. Nonetheless, since there is no rational guideline or framework by which to judge which vitamin or doses to use and for how long, how can anyone expect to reproduce alleged clinical success, let alone set up treatment plans coordinating megavitamin therapy with other modes of treatment?

Dr. Pauling carefully points out that orthomolecular medicine goes beyond the usual bounds of nutrition. That is, orthomolecular medicine, as he advocates it, uses nutrition and nutrients such as vitamins in a way they have never before been used. (No one disagrees with this.) He believes that, practiced correctly, orthomolecular medicine will probably cause little harm to the patient, and "quite possibly a great deal of good will result." Should such prospects and hope be the basis of therapy for illnesses such as schizophrenia? Pauling and his fellow advocates believe so, since they are not convinced that the usual philosophy and methods of treating mental illness are very successful. "This new, orthomolecular approach brings us new hope," he states. On the other hand, equally trained and knowledgable individuals believe that the real advances in this area are being made with the use of specific new synthetic agents that are the bulwark of what is called psychopharmacology (the science of using selected drugs in the management of mental illness).

A critical rationalization—and it is a particularly good one—of the proponents of orthomolecular medicine is that there is no such thing as the average human, let alone a typical patient with mental illness. That is, they wish to emphasize the individual. Of course, no one denies this as a valid objective in the treatment of any patient for any disease. There is abundant evidence that each person is biochemically, anatomically (and probably in other ways) unique and extraordinary. This idea has been elegantly promoted by the nutritionist-scientist Dr. Roger Williams (see Primary Sources). Is this good reason for the orthomolecular advocates to explain why they cannot give any standard treatment plan or schedule for general trial and scrutiny by their peers? Treatment evaluation techniques must be devised. Whether or not such techniques or methods will be accepted remains to be answered. Until then, the advocates of the rationale and success of orthomolecular medicine continue to describe their results in a manner somewhat between pure anecdotal accounts and pure double-blind–controlled studies.

There are other elements in the orthomolecular debate. Dr. Pauling convincingly argues that physicians have long used orthomolecular medicine without actually calling it such. Thus, he points out, when insulin is used to treat diabetes (abnormally high blood sugar), or iodine is used to prevent goiter (a malfunction of the thyroid gland that makes thyroid hormone), or fluoridation is used to help prevent tooth decay, these substances are being used to correct or straighten out abnormal cellular function or deficiencies. What he fails to mention, however, is that in each instance we know the exact role of insulin, iodine, and fluoride in the condition for which they are used. We know that the diabetic or goiter patient has a deficiency of these vital substances, and we can correct the condition to high degree by administering small amounts of the substance near that which would usually be seen in normal individuals. Megadoses of insulin or iodine are not required. Analogously, if mental illness is due to a deficiency of certain vitamins or other natural substances, may not these disturbances be corrected by the administration of these vitamins that are so demonstrably effective in small amounts? The orthomolecular answer to this question is that no one knows precisely the extent of the defect in vitamin metabolism (even if it were to exist in mental illness). Therefore, massive doses are needed rather than the usual remedial doses, as in the case of insulin in diabetes. Dr. Pauling argues that through possible gene mutations some individuals who may be particularly prone to certain diseases may require as much as a thousandfold increase in the required substance (e.g., a vitamin) in order to prevent or correct the disease. Do we have any good or convincing laboratory evidence of such a thousand fold increase in Vitamin B requirements in certain individuals who have symptoms of schizophrenia? The answer is no. Yet if the megavitamin therapy appears to be beneficial in any given person, this is taken as circumstantial evidence that a vitamin deficiency did exist at the onset. So go the circuitous arguments for and against this controversial aspect of medicine.

Individualized therapy notwithstanding, is there any constant factor or factors that the advocates of orthomolecular medicine and psychiatry use in the substantial majority of cases? Early treatment plans included niacin (Vitamin B_3), usually in combination with other modes of therapy such as electroshock. Review of the latest treatment regimens does not reveal this constant Vitamin B_3 element, however. Thus, over a period of approximately fifteen years, the orthomolecular therapists have modified their treatment plan. This has led many to believe there cannot be any rationality to their therapy, since it is constantly changing.

Regardless of the merits or detractions of the megavitamin therapy approach to certain illnesses, one thing remains abundantly clear to us: We feel it would be a great error for a person to diagnose his own illness and decide to treat it with megavitamin therapy using the over-the-counter, high-potency vitamin preparations that are available. Hypervitaminosis (toxicity resulting from excessive vitamins) is a real threat. Orthomolecular medicine, particularly as it uses megadoses of vitamins, must be considered at this time an experimental, unproven, and potentially dangerous form of therapy, for any disease.

III

VITAMINS IN SPECIAL CIRCUMSTANCES

Pregnancy

Pregnancy imposes special nutritional and vitamin demands, some of which are met by a normal, healthy diet, and some of which require supplementation. The Committee on Maternal Nutrition of the National Academy of Sciences recommends that excessive weight control diets *not* be imposed on pregnant women. The ideal is a 20 to 25 pound weight gain during pregnancy; this allows for proper nutrition of both mother and fetus and results in more healthy babies.

The increased vitamin demands are reflected in the 1974 RDA (see Appendix). Even a normal diet will probably not meet the requirements for iron, and so supplementary iron (30 to 60 milligrams per day) is recommended. Folic acid (see Glossary) supplements (200 to 400 micrograms per day) are also required, and the salt ingested should be iodized.

In a large group of women studied by S. Heller and colleagues (see Primary Sources), 40 to 60 percent of the women with uncomplicated pregnancies were suboptimally supplied with Vitamin B_6. They thus suggested that diet supplementation with Vitamin B_6 is advisable.

The concentrations of water-soluble vitamins are generally higher in the fetal blood than in maternal blood. This is especially true for thiamine, riboflavin, pyridoxine, folic acid, and Vitamins B_{12} and C. The placenta contains particularly high concentrations of vitamin B_{12} and folic acid, thus apparently acting as a reservoir of these substances. The lipid-soluble vitamins (see Glossary), on the contrary, are in approximately equal concentrations in maternal and fetal blood. The Vitamin A concentration of fetal blood is, in fact, somewhat lower than maternal blood.

Pregnancy is one of the situations in which vitamin supplementation of the normal, healthy diet is clearly advisable. However, caution is in order: Too much can do harm. For example, babies born of mothers on high doses of Vitamin B_6 may have excessively high B_6 requirements, and if these are not met, serious problems could develop in the infant.

Infancy and Childhood

Few vitamin problems occur in the breast-fed infant of a well-nourished mother, but Vitamin D intake may be low in some of these infants. The Vitamin A content of the cholostrum secreted during the three days after birth is much higher (600 I.U. per 100 milliliters) than maternal milk (70 I.U. per 100 milliliters), and thus the newborn receives an adequate reserve of Vitamin A. Deficiency diseases are not common in infants in the United States, but mild Vitamin K deficiencies occur. Scurvy due to Vitamin C deficiencies continues to be reported, especially in certain geographical areas such as the Southeast (including Florida, the Orange State). Vitamin D and folic acid deficiencies also occur.

Infants on formulas are subject to vitamin deficiencies. Cow's milk is low in Vitamin C. Goat's milk is comparable in folic acid content to cow's milk while providing less Vitamin B_{12}. Thus, infants fed goat's milk exclusively are likely to develop megaloblastic anemia, which responds better to folic acid therapy than to therapy with Vitamin B_{12}. An important source of vitamin loss is the heating of the formula. Vitamin B_6 is easily destroyed by heat. Vitamin E may be low when milk formulas are used. Commercially available formulas generally take these factors into consideration and include vitamin supplements.

As the carbohydrate content of the diet increases, so does the requirement for thiamine. Similarly, increase in protein intake is paralleled by an increased need for Vitamin B_6, while the pantothenic acid requirements decrease. An increased dietary intake of polyunsaturated fats results in increased requirements for Vitamin E. The composition of the diet influences the production of B vitamins by the microorganisms in the intestines, but whether these vitamins are then absorbed to a sufficient extent to be of practical value is uncertain.

Infants and children are more sensitive to vitamin deficiencies than adults. Comparable periods of deficiency produce far more serious effects in children. It is thus extremely important to supply adequate levels of vitamins, primarily by adequate diet and fortified milk.

Vitamin supplements for children have certainly been abused. S. Fomon (see Primary Sources) points out that the hazards of Vitamin A overdosage exceed the dangers of deficiencies. In fact, the reports of Vitamin A intoxication outnumber the reports of deficiency.

Studies have shown that 400 I.U. of Vitamin D per day is necessary for children from infancy through adolescence. However, due to the sensitivity of some infants and children to high doses of Vitamin D, the American Academy of Pediatrics has suggested that the Vitamin D enrichment of foods other than milk be discontinued.

Aging and Geriatrics

Old persons are particularly vulnerable to vitamin deficiencies. At a symposium on "Vitamins in the Elderly," held at the Royal College of Physicians in London, the reasons for this were discussed. These include: ignorance, social isolation, depression, poverty, physical disability, mental impairment, adverse social circumstances. The diet (and thus the vitamin intake) is least satisfactory in the mentally confused. Deficiencies in the elderly are most likely to include the B complex, C, and D vitamins. Two-thirds of those unable to look after themselves were found to be folate deficient (see Glossary).

Many elderly live in nursing homes, or spend long periods of time in hospitals. These persons may be more subject to vitamin deficiencies. Hospital food is often overcooked, and often long periods of time pass before the food is served. Donald Watkin (see Primary Sources) has been particularly interested in this area of nutrition. He noted from a study of hospital food in England that there usually was a nearly complete loss of Vitamin C in potatoes and a 75 percent loss in green vegetables. Since 30 percent of the national intake of Vitamin C (in England) is derived from potatoes, he was particularly concerned with the hospital management of this nutrient. He pointed out that a large percent of the Vitamin C content of potatoes is preserved if the potatoes are cooked and served in chunks, but the bulk of the potatoes served in English hospitals are mashed; mashing exposes the Vitamin C to air and thus virtually all the Vitamin C is destroyed.

A. Whanger (see Primary Sources) pointed out that in older persons the gastric secretions tend to inactivate thiamine, especially if hydrochloric acid is absent. Further changes in the bacterial content of the intestines in the elderly may inactivate thiamine. Diuretics, which a significant number of elderly take, increase the rate of excretion of thiamine.

Vitamin B_6 metabolism is altered in the elderly. The ability of the tissues to retain Vitamin C may decline with age. These are examples where age, in itself, may be a cause of vitamin deficiencies. But the associate causes, such as those mentioned above, are probably more important. Other associated causes include the fact that the elderly do not drink much milk, and often are not exposed to sunlight, and so may develop Vitamin D deficiencies.

Many chronic illnesses can lead to vitamin deficiencies: For example, liver diseases, biliary insufficiency, and uremia predispose to Vitamin K deficiencies. Further, the drugs taken by the elderly also may inactivate vitamins. To continue with the Vitamin K deficiency example, chronic use of antibiotics (by altering or destroying intestinal bacteria), the use of mineral oil for constipation, and extended use of aspirin may lead to Vitamin K deficiencies. Other drug-vitamin interactions have been mentioned elsewhere in this book.

In general, throughout this book we have pointed out that well-balanced diets will, in most cases, prevent vitamin deficiencies. However, the elderly present a special case since so many of them do *not* have adequate diets. Thus, vitamin supplements may be particularly appropriate in this segment of the population. For example, W. Griffiths (see Primary Sources), at the London Symposium on Vitamins in the Elderly, concluded that "The difficulties of correcting Vitamin B and C deficiencies in long-term hospitalized elderly patients by alteration in the food intake is . . . so immense that the only solution is to give vitamin supplements in tablet form indefinitely." A. Whanger usually prescribes multivitamin supplements in his elderly patients. He considers that the potential benefit greatly outweighs any remotely possible complications of their use, in the moderate doses he prescribes. However, it is important to be certain that the individual does not have pernicious anemia, since taking folic acid (see Glossary) will prevent some early symptoms of the disease from appearing, but will *not* prevent the serious neurological complications from developing.

The question of the role of Vitamin E in altering the aging process is being extensively studied and debated. The careful investigations being reported are those involving controlled experiments using animals and isolated tissues and cells. The reader may have observed that we have tried to confine our survey and discussion to the uses and actions of vitamins as they pertain to the human organism. We have purposely excluded discussion of the extensive literature of the actions of vitamins on animals and other organisms, although we have mentioned some animal studies when appropriate. This is not to imply that animal studies and results are unimportant; on the contrary, we believe that most of our good solid evidence of the actions of vitamins on cellular functions is derived from carefully controlled laboratory studies involving animals or animal tissues. Needless to say, it would be difficult if not impossible to perform on humans the variety of controlled experiments that are done with animals. Thus, the question of whether or not Vitamin E deficiency or treatment can accelerate or retard the aging process has been studied in rats. This can be done because the diet and conditions can be controlled, and the life span of the rat is short enough (about two years) to allow attainment of answers in a reasonably short time. To conduct similar experiments on man would be fraught with moral, ethical, and scientific problems.

Nonetheless, responsible scientists are seriously considering the possibility that certain cellular changes seen in aging in man may be beneficially influenced by providing an additional dietary source of Vitamin E or other natural or synthetic anti-oxidant materials. It must be emphasized that this is theory, not proven fact. Much research is needed. Until the evidence is in, responsible individuals cannot properly advocate the use of Vitamin E as a proven anti-aging vitamin. Indeed, no vitamin or combination of vitamins has proven to have anti-aging properties in man.

Brain Function

Vitamin deficiencies have been shown to affect brain function. The most serious effects are noted when the vitamin deficiency accompanies severe malnutrition, but isolated vitamin deficiencies also can produce marked brain dysfunction, such as epileptic-type seizures.

Severe malnutrition and vitamin deficiency during early infancy, or during fetal life, can produce a permanent reduction in brain size, a decrease in the number of brain cells, and permanently reduced brain function and mental ability.

A deficiency of Vitamin B_6 can produce brain seizures if the deficiency occurs during an early stage of brain development. In babies whose diets provided only 60 percent of the necessary Vitamin B_6, a single injection of pyridoxine (a form of Vitamin B_6) can reverse many of the brain wave abnormalities within three minutes. One-third of the children with brain abnormalities studied by D. Raine (see Primary Sources) revealed evidence of abnormalities of tryptophan (see Glossary) metabolism characteristic of Vitamin B_6 deficiency.

Subnormal folate levels have been found in 27 to 91 percent of treated epilepsy (see Glossary) patients. E. Reynolds (see Primary Sources) has reported that the common epileptic inhibiting drugs reduce folate levels in the serum, blood cells and cerebral spinal fluid. However, a word of caution is in order here: Folic acid and its derivatives have significant convulsant properties and can reverse the anticonvulsant effects of the drugs. This seems to be another case where too little of a vitamin is bad, but too much of the same vitamin is also bad.

Vitamin D deficiencies have also been shown to affect brain function. S. Arnand and G. Stickler (see Primary Sources) have emphasized the fact that Vitamin D deficiency can produce seizure activity, and that it is usually difficult to diagnose. In fact, of a group of Vitamin D deficient infants, in none was Vitamin D deficiency the first diagnosis. Some were suspected of having epilepsy.

We have previously stated that it is often difficult to separate the symptoms of vitamin deficiencies and malnutrition. In the case of brain functions, another important element has to be considered. The amount of activity and the intellectual challenges that a child receives can also be important. Animal studies have revealed, for example, that environment enrichment can produce a considerably thicker brain cortex than occurs in environmental impoverishment. Furthermore, the total brain weight, the development of brain cells and the contacts between brain cells are also affected. These studies have been more extensively discussed by one of us (Paul Bach-y-Rita) in a previous book (see Primary Sources).

The effects of vitamin deficiencies on brain functions are often indirect. For example, listlessness and general poor health can lead to poor school performance and lack of participation in an active life, which is the equivalent of "environmental impoverishment" in the animal studies. The Committee on International Nutrition Programs has stated that ". . . the existent studies suggest that anemia in the preschool years adversely affects motivation and ability to concentrate for extended periods of time." Anemia can be caused by malnutrition, or by specific vitamin deficiencies, such as folic acid and Vitamin B_{12} deficiencies.

The effect of vitamins on mental illness is a current area of interest. Although several research groups have found megavitamin therapy to be of use, others do not and the task force report of the Psychiatric Association concluded that no usefulness has been demonstrated. However, vitamin deficiencies may cause mental symptoms. Some have been mentioned above. Further, thiamine deficiency in alcoholics has been associated with hallucinations. Confusional states in the elderly have been related to vitamin deficiencies. In some women taking oral contraceptives (see Glossary), Vitamin B_6 deficiencies appear to be associated with depression; in such cases studied by P. Adams et al. (see Primary Sources), administration of Vitamin B_6 improved the mental status.

IS VITAMIN B_{12} A SAFE TONIC?

The average daily requirement for adult men and women for Vitamin B_{12} has been established at 3 micrograms per day. As little as 0.5 to 1 microgram per day given by injection has been shown to be effective in controlling pernicious anemia (see Glossary), the main disease that results from B_{12} deficiency.

Despite this remarkable potency and the specificity of the disease response, it is commonly held that vitamin B_{12} supplements may be beneficial in treating nervous disorders and poorly defined fatigue and "rundown feelings." The average diet in the United States supplies, primarily through animal products, between 1 and 100 micrograms per day. (Obviously, vegetarians could show a true dietary deficiency of B_{12}, and supplementation might be required.) Then why do individuals and physicians resort to the use of B_{12} in amounts several hundred to a thousand times that which can be utilized by the body? At the most, pregnant women may require 4 micrograms per day.

It has been shown that these massive doses of B_{12} have no physiological action unless there is actually a deficiency. Then, it would respond to the much smaller amounts indicated. Several studies have now shown that in fact the apparent improvement of patients receiving injections of Vitamin B_{12} is psychological. That is, the mere procedure of receiving an injection by a physician is sufficient to affect the patient's apparent ills. This is the well-known placebo effect often seen in medicine. It is no better exemplified than in the cases of miraculous cures of fatigue and nervous conditions following injections of Vitamin B_{12}.

Another feature of Vitamin B_{12} that is often forgotten is that while injected microgram doses (that needed by the body) are readily retained by the body, the milligram doses that are often injected are rapidly excreted in the urine.

Weight Reduction

Vitamins have always had a prominent role in reducing diets and regimens. Perhaps this is good. Certainly if one is reducing caloric intake there is a strong possibility that certain normal vitamin intake will suffer as a result. Most "over-the-counter" diet aids boast of their vitamin-mineral content.

It should be kept in mind that vitamins have no calories in themselves. They serve as co-factors in vital cellular reactions. On the other hand, no single vitamin, or combination of vitamins, will, by themselves, "burn-up" calories. Thus, injections or ingestion of any single vitamin or combination of vitamins without any change in caloric intake cannot cause a reduction in weight. This is often misunderstood because of the claims of various reducing aids, but is clearly true.

Vitamin supplementation is not ordinarily essential in a diet plan, although this may depend on the vitamin stores in any individual. That is, it may depend upon how adequate a diet existed before weight reduction was started. However, prolonged dieting (one month or more) should, for safety, be supplemented with extra vitamins.

The purported cholesterol-lowering effect of lecithin in reducing diets has been debated and explored, and it finds no place in the modern armamentarium used to lower blood cholesterol.

Similarly, the use of B_6 as an agent to beneficially affect salt and water metabolism with the presumed effect on total body water finds no support in the extensive literature on the biological effects of B_6 (in the doses recommended in some regimens).

The success anyone may have on any reducing regimen is probably related to the required reduction in calorie intake. The fact that the regimen will not work without such caloric restriction is well known.

What is being spuriously advocated is that vitamins aid in the loss of weight and inches. Is such an argument sound enough for critical consumers who also may speak out against unethical advertisements promoting children's cereals, or empty nutrition, or inadequately labeled foods?

Oral Contraceptives

Some women taking The Pill may show a clear syndrome of mental depression. Physicians wondered about the reason for this apparent association of drug and symptoms. It is now thought that in some cases this depression may be the result of the drug inhibiting the synthesis of certain substances in the brain that are required for normal functioning of the central nervous system. It turns out that the synthesis of these substances (catecholamines) requires pyridoxine, and that the estrogen in the oral contraceptive results in a functional deficiency of this necessary vitamin. This depression might be prevented or reversed by the administration of supplemental amounts of Vitamin B_6. For example, in a group of depressed women taking oral contraceptives, whose symptoms were judged to be due to the oral contraceptives, P. Adams and co-workers (see Primary Sources) found B_6 deficiencies in eleven of the twenty-two cases studied. The B_6-deficient group responded clinically to B_6 administration, while the others did not.

In addition, women taking oral contraceptives may not have adequate stores of Vitamin B_6 to meet the increased demand for this vitamin during future pregnancies, when the dietary intake may be suboptimal due to voluntary food restriction for weight control.

There is a possibility, however, that Vitamin B_6 supplements to the diets of women taking oral contraceptives may diminish their reserves of amino acids. It is not known at present whether this is an important consideration.

Most medical attention has focused on the changes in Vitamin B_6 associated with the use of oral contraceptives. However, other important vitamin-oral contraceptive drug relationships are now being examined. For example, a recent report has shown that women taking oral contraceptive agents showed no significant changes in their blood Vitamin E or C levels. The most consistent changes noted were the elevation in Vitamin A and an increase in conversion of tryptophan to niacin. An increase in the chemical conversion of carotene (see Glossary) to Vitamin A was also likely. (Incidentally, serum copper levels were significantly and consistently elevated in the oral contraceptive group.) The rise in Vitamin A may be of some physiological consequence, especially to a fetus should a woman conceive soon after terminating oral contraceptive therapy.

Other investigators have found that a group of women taking oral contraceptives had elevated Vitamin E and A levels, but there was a lower level of folicin and Vitamin B_{12}. Obviously, oral contraceptives have a complex pharmacology and physiology. Certainly more research will be needed before it can be clearly determined what precautions, if any, should be taken regarding vitamin supplementation (or withdrawal?) in women taking these drugs.

Alcoholism

Alcohol has a high calorie content, and so the energy requirements of the body are supplied in this way by the heavy drinker. However, this results in nutritional and vitamin deficiencies, primarily because of decreased intake of foods that contain the essential nutrients and vitamins. In addition, other factors also must be considered: The alcoholic may have impaired vitamin absorption as well as increased requirements. For example, alcohol interferes with the intermediate metabolism of folic acid. Also, liver and pancreatic diseases produced by the alcoholism further modify the vitamin requirements. (See section on vitamins in relation to other substances.) And contrary to prevailing opinion, the content of B vitamins in American beer is so low as to have little nutritional value.

It is worth emphasizing here that thiamine deficiency is a common and very serious occurrence in alcoholism. It causes many peripheral and central nervous system disorders such as alcoholic neuritis. Prompt treatment with large doses of thiamine is thus initiated in the hospital when alcoholism is diagnosed.

The consumption of large amounts of alcohol (ethanol) by alcoholics carries risks that go beyond the well-documented effects on the liver and brain. It has now been shown that Vitamin A is an essential substance for the normal development of sperm. It has been found that alcohol inhibits the oxidation of Vitamin

A by testicular tissue. Vitamin A is oxidized to the active form (retinol) by the enzyme alcohol dehydrogenase (ADH). This enzyme metabolizes ethanol to acetaldehyde. (This enzyme is found in the retina of the eye as well as in testicular tissue.) Alcoholics may thus experience night blindness because of the competitive inhibition of retinol formation in the eye by the ingested alcohol. Similarly, a relative Vitamin A deficiency in testicular tissue may result from chronic ethanol consumption, with the effect that normal sperm production may be impaired, and sterility can result. The fact that 50 to 70 percent of male chronic alcoholics who show cirrhosis of the liver may also have impaired sperm production supports the biochemical evidence of a complex alcohol–Vitamin A interaction by the body.

Cancer

Although a general discussion of cancer is beyond the scope of this book, we considered it appropriate and necessary to deal with some of the controversies relating to the role of vitamins in the prevention or treatment of cancer. The very enigma of cancer —its causes, its effects, its prevention, its cure—has resulted in the emergence of many ideas and myths concerning the possible role and effects of vitamins in this dread disease. We shall review here some of these ideas and concepts in the hope that the reader will develop a critical perspective toward the many advocates (ethical and unethical) who see an essential role for vitamins in this disease.

Is there any convincing or compelling scientific evidence that cancer (in any of its many forms) may be due to a vitamin deficiency? This question is complex, but it probably can be answered no. This is not to say that the symptoms of certain kinds of cancers cannot be made worse by relative lack of certain vitamins. For example, the possibility has been discussed by Dr. Solomon Garb (see Primary Sources) that some of the symptoms occasionally seen in patients with leukemia (a form of blood cancer involving excessive production of certain white blood cells) may be due to the relative lack of Vitamin C. His argument is that the abnormal leukemia cells may take up large amounts of the available Vitamin C in the blood. This might cause a decrease in the amount of available vitamin to other tissues, with the result that the patient may begin to show the classic sign of Vitamin C deficiency, that is, scurvy (soft, spongy gums, bleeding tendency). Does administration of Vitamin C to such patients help eliminate these signs and symptoms? The question is certainly worthy of study. As Dr. Garb points out, there does appear to be a rationale for administering large doses of Vitamin C to such susceptible leukemia patients. These doses would assure that there would be an adequate blood level of the vitamin that otherwise could not be obtained since the leukemic cells may take up such large amounts of the vitamin.

The exact amount of Vitamin C that would have to be administered to correct the relative vitamin deficiency can be based upon precise measurement of the ascorbic acid levels in the blood and white cells. In leukemia, there may be as much as ten times the normal number of white cells, with a corresponding increase in the amount of ascorbic acid (Vitamin C) that they might take up. Dr. Garb has estimated that 5 grams of Vitamin C in divided doses should be sufficient to saturate the white cells and also provide adequate blood levels of the substance.

But this point must be emphasized: When and if such Vitamin C therapy or treatment is used in leukemia, the cancer per se is not being treated or cured. It is only the *symptoms* of the relative ascorbic acid deficiency that are being treated. The patient would obviously be better off not suffering symptoms of Vitamin C deficiency in addition to the other medical effects of the blood cancer. The vitamin deficiency is being treated, not the cancer. The layman should be clear on this point.

This example raises the broader question of the general uses of other vitamins in other forms of cancer. One cannot deny that it is good medical practice to maintain an adequate nutritional state in the cancer patient. This may be particularly important in those forms of cancer where there is poor appetite, abnormal bowel function, or unusual metabolic demands (resulting from surgery or anticancer drugs) that alter the normal requirements for vitamins and other essential nutrients. In patients who are unable to meet their regular metabolic needs for vitamins and other nutrients, it is advisable to administer supplemental doses of those vitamins and other nutrients that are suspected of being deficient. Moreover, radiation (or X-ray) treatment of cancer often causes great disturbances in the patient's nutritional demands. Adjunctive therapy with vitamins and other essential nutrients might be used to maintain some semblance of nutritional well-being. Such supplemental vitamin therapy might also be applied to the patient who will undergo or has undergone surgery for cancer. Because of the stress of such surgery, some surgeons utilize some vitamin-nutritional support therapy to aid the patient's recovery or enhance the healing process. In acute cases, short-term infusions of multivitamins are often used. (The direct infusion of vitamins through a vein also may be used in other conditions where the physician suspects that a nutritional deficiency may be the result of surgery, burns, fractures, infectious diseases, trauma, coma, etc.). In such patients, administration of multivitamin preparations containing Vitamin C (500 mg), Vitamin A (10,000 USP units), Vitamin D (ergocalciferol) (1,000 USP units), thiamine (B_1) (50 mg), riboflavin (B_2) (10 mg), pyridoxine (B_6) (15 mg), niacinamide (100 mg) and Vitamin E (25 mg) might be helpful in the medical management of the primary disease state. (These solutions are not injected directly; they are diluted with physiological salt solution containing saline, dextrose, or other infusion solutions.)

Again, this must be emphasized: The primary disease of cancer is not being treated or cured with such vitamin therapy. The patient is receiving nutritional support in a condition where experience suggests there may be need for adjunctive therapy. This is just another aspect in the total management of the cancer patient that might be used to restore a more normal physiological state that would otherwise be deteriorating as the result of the disease or as a result of other forms of treatment used to combat the cancer (e.g., X-ray therapy, surgery). On the other hand, physicians must be on the alert for possible worsening caused by vitamins in certain types of cancers. A case in point is Vitamin D. In some forms of cancer, there is an excess of calcium in the blood. Drugs that decrease this calcium level are important in managing such patients. On the other hand, administration of Vitamin D, which may raise blood calcium levels, may aggravate the primary calcium disorder related to the presence of malignant disease.

Another aspect of vitamin therapy in cancer should be emphasized. This relates to the placebo effect of administering medication to a sick patient. Cancer patients often have little hope of any substantial "cure" for their disease. The more the physician does for them, the more confidence the patient has that *something* is being tried. Many cancer patients (and others as well) receive substantial benefit from "that vitamin shot the doctor gave me," even though the vitamin in itself may not produce any meaningful change in the disease state.

So far we have emphasized the potential use of vitamins in the general nutritional support of the cancer patient. Is there any evidence that a cancer patient may benefit from an induced vitamin deficiency?

Drs. Gailani, Ohnuma, and Rosen (see Primary Sources) have neatly summarized this aspect of potential cancer treatment. They point out there may indeed be some rationale for treating some forms of cancer by inducing a deficiency of vitamins. This strategy is based on the fact that vitamins are constituents of vital cell components such as coenzymes (see Glossary) which are essential molecules needed for cell growth and function. If one were to deprive the growing cancer cell of such vital elements, then cancer growth and spread might be impaired. (Here it is assumed that the cancer cell has an unusual requirement for these vitamin-containing coenzymes. Normal cells may have less of a demand for maintenance of their function.) Based upon these considerations, riboflavin deficiency has been induced in humans suffering from cancer. Deficiency of this vitamin was brought about by diet restriction of the vitamin plus use of a specific drug that antagonized the normal actions of riboflavin. In such riboflavin-deficient patients, manifestations of the vitamin deficiency were seen. In two patients, there was transient improvement in their clinical status, and one patient showed minor tumor regression. Similar trials were tried with Vitamin B_6

depletion. No antitumor effect was seen. There appears to be a similar lack of effectiveness in human cancer when nicotinamide deficiency is induced.

In general, therefore, there is no firm clinical evidence to suggest a major beneficial role for inducing vitamin-deficient states in man for the treatment of cancer.

Some promising lines of research relating vitamins to cancer should be mentioned.

Folate (see Glossary) antagonists may have a role in the treatment of certain cancers. Richard Rivlin (see Primary Sources), in a review of these studies, has stated: "Not only do vitamins affect the rate of neoplastic growth, but tumors, in turn, may affect the metabolism of vitamins. Vitamins also affect the inactivation of drugs and may influence the response to chemotherapy."

One vitamin has been receiving wide attention in several cancer research centers for its potential effect in protecting the body from harmful substances that may cause cancer (carcinogens). The research suggests that Vitamin A and its derivatives may be potential mediators of interference of cell transformation that is an effect of certain carcinogens.

Vitamin A (retinol) has long been known to influence the differentiation of certain cells into more specialized tissues. The clue that was important to the researchers is that many of the carcinogens produce their damaging effect in lower than normal amounts in animals that have Vitamin A deficiency (i.e., the carcinogenic effect is enhanced). Even in animals that are not deprived of this vitamin and are then exposed to the cancer-producing substance, administration of additional quantities of the vitamin can produce a protective effect. The beneficial action of the vitamin in these experiments is not fully understood. One suggestion, based on laboratory evidence, is that the vitamin may stimulate the immune response of the animals, and this offers protection against the carcinogen insult.

While these results are encouraging to the scientist, they and others who read the results are fearful that the *potential* of this kind of therapy or treatment will be a stimulus for the cancer and nutritional faddists to begin Vitamin A treatment for the prevention of cancer in man. In fact, the extrapolated amounts of the vitamin needed in humans probably would precipitate severe Vitamin A toxicity. (Synthetic analogs of the vitamin may get around this difficulty.) In the meantime, everyone involved with such research cautions against the use of available Vitamin A as an anticancer agent. Such self-medication is dangerous, and even if applied to human needs tomorrow, would be under the strictest medical and scientific control. We cite this example since so much of the good scientific research on vitamins, even though preliminary in nature and offering some potential benefits, is pounced upon by cancer and nutritional faddists before all the required information is in. Do not be misguided by these opportunists. There are already too many quack cancer cures.

IV

FREQUENTLY OVERLOOKED FACTORS

Vitamins in Relation to Other Substances

Physicians who prescribe, or individuals who buy, vitamins usually think of how each vitamin being consumed is producing the desired effect. Rare consideration is given to the interrelationship or interaction of one vitamin with another or with other substances. This is an important feature of vitamins that is often overlooked by professionals and laymen alike.

For example, a good understanding of Vitamin A interaction with other vitamins is now available. Research has indicated that consumption of Vitamin E may affect the utilization of Vitamin A. This interaction depends upon the amount of unsaturated fatty acids (see Glossary) (e.g., corn oil) and carotene in the diet. This is illustrated by the fact that as little as 5 to 10 mg of alpha-tocopherol (Vitamin E) per day may be needed by normal men consuming low amounts of linoleic acid. However, the prolonged ingestion of large amounts of vegetable oils (as often advocated for the prevention of heart disease) may increase the requirement of Vitamin E threefold to sixfold.

Theoretically, as the body oxidizes Vitamin E, the product can be chemically reduced back to its natural (biologically active) tocopherol form by the presence of Vitamin C, which might serve as an antioxidant chemical.

The way Vitamin A is metabolized by the body depends on the presence of Vitamin D.

Consumption of large amounts of Vitamin C (as often advocated for the prevention or treatment of the common cold) may preserve the function of chemically reduced folates. Similarly, chemical studies suggest that ascorbic acid also may protect thiamine, riboflavin, and pantothenic acid from being oxidized in the body.

Vitamin C has been shown to have important interactions with commonly used drugs. For example, administration of 500 mg of Vitamin C to humans has been reported to interact with simultaneously ingested aspirin. One to three aspirin tablets (300 to 900 mg of drug) given to normal male subjects will cause a significant elevation of the amount of Vitamin C in blood plasma resulting from prior administration of 500 mg of the vitamin. The degree of elevation of the plasma level of the vitamin depended upon the amount of aspirin taken. However, the amount of Vitamin C found in white blood cells (leucocytes) of the same subjects did not change from the levels found prior to taking two aspirin tablets. It was also found that taking aspirin does not interfere with absorption of Vitamin C from the gastrointestinal tract. Apparently the presence of aspirin in the blood competes with Vitamin C storage in the white blood cells, with the result that there is a diminished storage of ascorbic acid in the leucocyte. Thus, the usual therapeutic dose of two aspirin tablets inhibits the normal uptake of Vitamin C by an important storage site in the body, namely the white blood cells. It would appear that people who must take aspirin on a regular basis (for example, arthritic patients) should perhaps increase their Vitamin C intake to assure adequate levels of Vitamin C in their white blood cells, since the amount of vitamin excreted by the kidneys is increased by the presence of aspirin.

On the other hand, it is well known that high doses of ascorbic acid may so acidify the urine that patients who are taking salicylate drugs such as aspirin will have increased blood levels of the drug due to the fact there is an increased reabsorption of the drug by the kidneys. Thus, caution must be used by those who are taking large doses of Vitamin C along with high doses of a salicylate (e.g., 3 to 5 grams per day). Other anti-inflammatory drugs such as indomethacin and phenylbutazone may inhibit the normal metabolism of Vitamin C by the body.

A clinically harmful and dangerous effect of megadoses of folic acid (folate) has been described in epileptics who have been receiving drug therapy for their disease. Since drugs like diphenylhydantoin (Dilantin) used in the treatment of epilepsy may cause a lowering of serum folate, some investigators felt that intravenous administration of the folate would correct the drug-induced disturbance. Patients receiving 75 mg of folate intravenously varied in their responses to the injections. In some patients there was no discernible clinical effect. Others, even when given lower doses, showed abnormalities of their brain electrical patterns and went into outright seizures. It was concluded that even though there is some uniformity in the epileptic population receiving Dilantin therapy in regard to reduced serum folate levels, their response to large doses of the vitamin are less predictable; consequently megadoses of the vitamin must be used with great caution in such conditions.

Other complex drug-vitamin interactions are possible. Take the case of children or adults with epilepsy or other convulsant disorders. Patients who are taking anticonvulsant drugs such as diphenylhydantoin or barbiturates may develop classic sign of Vitamin D deficiency, i.e., rickets. This is due to the fact that these drugs may destroy Vitamin D. By administering large doses of Vitamin D to such patients rickets is prevented.

A recent report in the *Journal of the American Medical Association* (230:241, 1974) has pointed out the potential dangers of excessive Vitamin C consumption on the utilization or function of Vitamin B_{12}. It was reported that a low dose of Vitamin C (0.1 gram) had no significant effect on the Vitamin B_{12} content of meals high in B_{12}. However, if there was only a moderate amount of Vitamin B_{12} present, 43 percent of the Vitamin B_{12} was destroyed. A higher amount of ascorbic acid (0.25 gram) destroyed 81 percent of the Vitamin B_{12} in the meal containing moderate amounts of B_{12}, and 25 percent was destroyed in the high Vitamin B_{12} content meal. A still higher concentration of Vitamin C (0.5 gram) destroyed an amazing 95 percent of the Vitamin B_{12} in the moderate B_{12} meal, and almost 50 percent was destroyed by ascorbic acid even when Vitamin B_{12} was present in large amounts. There is no evidence to suggest that the daily adult RDA dose of Vitamin C (30 to 45 mg) destroys Vitamin B_{12} in food.

These interesting results point to the strong possibility that there might be a great nutritional consequence of taking high doses of Vitamin C on the availability of Vitamin B_{12} normally available in meals. The degree of inactivation of B_{12} by ascorbic acid not only depends on the amount of Vitamin C present but on the amount of B_{12} present in the different meals. It is likely that the destruction of Vitamin B_{12} in food would be less extensive, if at all, if the Vitamin C were taken several hours after consumption of the meal.

Vitamin B_{12} is needed by the body for certain chemical reactions in which the substance folate (folic acid or folacin) serves as a coenzyme in cell function. In addition, a Vitamin B_{12} deficiency that might result from the described interactions with ascorbic acid may result in altered chemical reactions involving carbohydrates, fat, and protein.

In contrast to the destructive action of Vitamin C on B_{12}, it is known that Vitamin C may have a chemically protective effect on the B complex vitamins such as thiamine and riboflavin, as well as on vitamins A and E.

One of the popular beliefs concerning the virtues of high doses of Vitamin C is that it may reduce blood cholesterol levels. Lowering of blood cholesterol has been deemed an important goal in American nutrition, at least from the pronouncements of the American Heart Association and various national health agencies. It is therefore interesting to note the study of a research group in Nairobi, Kenya. They studied some pastoral tribes in Kenya who had a high cholesterol dietary intake. Their blood cholesterol was measured, along with the ascorbic acid content of their blood white cells (leukocytes), a major storage depot for the vitamin. These researchers found that the higher the blood serum level of cholesterol, the higher the Vitamin C content of the blood white blood cells. Particularly in the Masai and Turkana tribes, it was observed that low serum cholesterol levels were associated with low ascorbic acid content of the leucocytes. Their findings indicate support for the notion that under conditions of high dietary cholesterol intake, serum cholesterol level is proportionate to ascorbic acid levels. The implications of such research to problems of prevention or treatment of atherosclerosis remain obscure, however. One thing appears clear, however: According to recently published studies from Stanford University, consumption for two months of 4 grams per day of Vitamin C by patients with elevated blood levels of cholesterol does not result in any significant change in plasma cholesterol or major fatty substances (triglycerides). There thus appears to be no scientific basis for the promotion of ascorbic acid as a natural means for reducing blood cholesterol levels, especially in patients with elevated blood cholesterol.

Other substances may interact with vitamins in foods. Many common food additives may thus adversely affect the content of vitamins in meat and milk, for example. Two cases in point may be cited: Sulphur dioxide, once used as a food treatment, may decrease the thiamine content of meat and milk. On the other hand, the formation of potentially dangerous nitrosamines from nitrites (which are sometimes used as chemical preservatives in certain foods such as meats) can be prevented by the presence of adequate amounts of ascorbic acid, which probably functions as an antioxidant. Laboratory studies have shown that sodium nitrite, sodium nitrate, and sodium citrate, commonly used as food additives, may cause a considerable decrease in the thiamine, riboflavin, and Vitamin C content of foods stored for fifteen, thirty, or forty-five days. This loss of vitamin activity was not seen when the food additives were absent.

Vitamin B_6–drug interactions are sometimes seen in patients who are taking the drug levodopa for Parkinson's syndrome (tremor). It is now well established that this vitamin reverses the beneficial effects of the drug in this disease. Doses as small as 10 to 25 mg of Vitamin B_6 may be sufficient to cancel out the desired effect of levodopa on brain function. It is now cautioned that individuals taking this drug should not take vitamin preparations containing Vitamin B_6. In fact, one of the manufacturers of levodopa now promotes a vitamin preparation devoid of Vitamin B_6 which can be taken by the patient who is on levodopa therapy.

Another caution about vitamin interactions with other substances must be stated: Many vitamins can interfere with important laboratory tests that are used by physicians in diagnosing illness. Most clinical laboratories are aware of these interferences of laboratory tests caused by certain vitamins. They are usually careful to question the patient who comes in for a blood or urine test about that patient's use of vitamin supplements. Several common examples may be given to illustrate this feature of vitamin use.

Vitamin C, by virtue of its ability to act as a chemical reducing substance, may cause a falsely high value of uric acid in the blood, if the uric acid test is not done by the enzymatic method. This interference of uric acid determination does not ordinarily occur when RDA amounts of the vitamin are being taken. Very recent evidence suggests Vitamin C tablets are oxidized in the bottle. This may contribute to the high uric acid readings in blood tests.

Large doses of riboflavin may cause a yellow discoloration of the urine that may be misleading to the clinical pathologist if he is not advised of the fact the vitamin is being taken. The B complex vitamins also may cause fluorescent substances to be excreted in the urine, and these may interfere with the determination of certain chemicals in the urine.

Vitamin C also may have some significance in drug addicts. A recent clinical report indicates that plasma and tissue ascorbic acid levels in seemingly healthy drug addicts were reduced to deficiency levels in 58 percent of the patients measured. The possible role of drug-related ascorbic acid deficiency in producing some of the symptoms of drug abuse are interesting to speculate about.

Since some vitamins such as ascorbic acid, particularly in doses used in megavitamin therapy, may affect the metabolism of some drugs, it is of more than theoretical interest to suggest that accurate measurement of drug levels in blood and urine may be interfered with. Thus, certain drugs must be carefully monitored in patients by actually determining the amount of the parent drug or its metabolites in body fluids such as blood, plasma, serum, or urine. If a vitamin, such as ascorbic acid, alters the way in which the body handles or excretes these drugs, then a spurious drug value will be obtained. Besides the laboratory consideration is the fact that humans, particularly those having a deficiency or excess of certain vitamins involved in the cellular metabolism of drugs, may show changed sensitivity to drug effects (e.g., reduced action or enhanced toxicity). Of particular concern would be the case of an individual who requires addition of Vitamin C supplements because of a demonstrated need of this vitamin. How long does it take him to re-establish adequate or normal drug metabolism after initiation of the vitamin supplements or upon withdrawal of the vitamin?

One can only conclude from these complex facts and observations that people who take vitamins should be aware that these substances may interact with a variety of other substances. Individuals who take drugs, obtained either by prescription or over-the-counter, should be extremely cautious about the promiscuous use of vitamins. The complex reactions that can occur may cause either a cancellation of the beneficial effects of drug or vitamin or an increase in the toxicity of drug or vitamin. Reports are being published monthly of such interactions of vitamins with other substances. This book cannot survey all of the evidence at this time. However, a word to the wise: Consult your physician before you take *any* drugs and vitamins, especially on a regular basis.

Vitamin Dependency

Large doses of vitamins may have another negative effect: They may cause dependency. William Darby (see Primary Sources) discusses the pyridoxine-dependent syndrome. It has been suggested that the sudden withdrawal of Vitamin C could create a more serious potential side effect than could urine acidity; plasma levels dropped to well below pretreatment levels for a period of ten to fourteen days following discontinuation. Robert Hodges (see Primary Sources) suggests that a pregnant woman who consumes massive doses of Vitamin C could bear a child with a Vitamin C dependency syndrome.

Placebo Effects

Many people take vitamins because it makes them "feel good" or gives them "more energy" or because it keeps them from getting colds or some other illness. It is extremely difficult to argue with these subjective impressions. It is also difficult to design scientific studies to test these impressions. Darby (see Primary Sources) has reviewed several studies that attempted to determine whether these subjective responses were due to a real action of the vitamin or to the power of suggestion (Placebo effect), and in conclusion he stated: "The non-specific general tonic-like effect commonly attributed to [vitamin] supplements is merely a placebo effect." He has further stated: "From time to time suggestions have been put forth that various ill-understood conditions appear to respond to massive quantities of one or another vitamin. These suggestions have usually followed within a relatively short time the recognition of the clinical usefulness of a vitamin in a deficiency disease." He considers this "wishful thinking." The pharmacologists Louis Goodman and Alfred Gillman (see Primary Sources) reflect the conclusion of many scientists that "the vitamins often represent nothing more than expensive placebos."

These conclusions are undoubtedly correct. However, the power of suggestion is very real. Thus, if a person is firmly convinced that he will "feel better" if he takes a certain vitamin, he will. This power of suggestion may also extend to certain disease states. The firm conviction that one is improving and recovering has a strong influence on the recovery. One of us (Paul Bach-y-Rita) had an opportunity to observe these effects during a period as a public health officer and a practicing physician in a remote region of Southern Mexico. Most of the medical problems were attended to by medicine men and witch doctors. Their methods were primitive and without scientific foundation but they often *worked.*

Although some useful drugs (such as digitoxin and reserpine) have emerged from folk medicine, most of the "medicines" so developed do not survive a controlled clinical test. However, placebos were useful in this remote practice, especially in view of the cultural heritage of the population. Modern medicine is learning to accept these nonscientifically based methods as having some basis in fact: It appears that the mind does have an element of control over body functions and reactions.

Therefore, a placebo effect cannot be dismissed as trivia. Vitamins definitely have many real functions in human biology, discussed throughout this book, as well as some very real pharmacological effects. However, a rational evaluation of vitamins must lead to the conclusion that many of the apparently miraculous effects claimed for vitamins are a result of the power of suggestion, and that any other substance that could inspire as much faith would have similar effects.

It should be emphasized that the placebo effect may not even require the use of "sugar pills" in the usual context. Thus, Stewart Wolf (see Primary Sources) has defined a placebo as "any effect attributed to a pill, potion, or procedure, but not to its pharmacodynamic or specific properties." Hence, variables affecting response of patients include treatment settings (e.g., the doctor's office), presence of others (e.g., nurse personnel or laboratory technicians), professional communication with the patient, the type of treatment, and the type of medication (or "sugar pill"), including its color, taste, and route of administration. In addition, the physician's or health professional's personality, optimism, enthusiasm, sympathy, authoritarianism, and demonstrated faith in the treatment plan can influence patient responses independent of any actually measured biological action of the procedure or drug.

Most studies involving placebo controls now indicate that 30 to 50 percent of those tested may be placebo reactors. This is significant, since in order to show any efficacy with any treatment plan (e.g., the benefits of Vitamin E in heart disease) it would be necessary to demonstrate that the plan was significantly better than the placebo response. This is why the FDA demands such strict control of drug experiments. It is interesting to note that the same scrutiny does not apply normally to the multitude of claims concerning vitamins. In fact, some investigators feel that the FDA is using a double standard, and they should in fact begin to control and regulate the studies of the effects of vitamins and the many exaggerated claims that fill our advertisements and popular reading material.

Vitamin Toxicity

If some vitamin supplementation is good, more is better; right? *Wrong.* Too much can be dangerous and harmful. In general, excesses of the fat-soluble vitamins are more difficult for the body to get rid of than the water-soluble vitamins, but some of the latter may also cause problems.

Too much of a vitamin may have the opposite effect than just enough of it. For example, whereas 300 to 400 I.U. of Vitamin D daily leads to maximum retention of calcium and phosphorous, the use of 1,800 I.U. or more daily for several months *decreases* the appetite and as a consequence *reduces* the total retentions of calcium and phosphorous and slows linear growth.

When vitamins are taken in the "recommended" amounts required to prevent diseases associated with vitamin deficiency (scurvy, rickets, beriberi, etc.), they do not generally cause toxic or adverse effects on the body. However, the Federal Food and Drug Administration's National Clearinghouse for Poison Control Centers reports that approximately 4,000 cases of documented vitamin poisonings occur each year; about 80 percent of the cases involve children. Of course, these statistics reveal only those cases of toxicity that usually require emergency medical treatment or hospitalization. Unknown numbers of vitamin users also experience signs and symptoms of vitamin toxicity or overdosage, but these go unreported. Thus, skin rashes, diarrhea, muscle cramps, kidney malfunction, and a variety of other complaints occur as the result of vitamin overindulgence. The unwary sufferer of these vitamin overdose symptoms probably will not relate the disorder to injudicious use of vitamins. Indeed, he may resort to taking *more* vitamins in the misbelief that the body disorder is the result of too few vitamins rather than too many.

B. Frame and his colleagues (see Primary Sources) have reported three interesting cases of excessive Vitamin A intake, one in a seven-year-old, another in a sixteen-year-old, and the third in a forty-six-year-old vitamin salesman. They have also pointed out that in many multivitamin preparations, both Vitamin A and Vitamin D may be present in amounts larger than the daily recommended dose. Excessive calcium accumulation in the body as well as bone changes may be caused by the combined effects of the two vitamins. Furthermore, some persons have a higher sensitivity to Vitamins A and D, and such persons will show signs of hypervitaminosis (see Glossary) with lower doses than in normal persons.

The seven-year-old patient reported by B. Frame and his collaborators entered the hospital with generalized muscular and skeletal discomfort, inability to straighten his legs, headache, irritability, and poor appetite. It turned out that he had been taking too much Vitamin A for two years, but that because of poor appetite, his parents doubled the Vitamin A intake *on the advice of a salesman in a health food store.* The sixteen-year-old at first denied taking vitamin supplements, but when confronted with the evidence admitted that he wanted to become an aircraft pilot, and hoping to improve his vision, he had taken too much Vitamin A for several years. The forty-six-year-old vitamin salesman also denied taking excessive amounts of Vitamin A, but intensive questioning finally resulted in an admission. His strong denial of excessive vitamin use delayed by many months the initiation of effective treatment. Furthermore, after the appearance of the first symptoms he had increased the dose, thinking that his symptoms indicated a need for larger amounts of nutritional supplements.

Vitamin D taken in excessive doses can cause mental and physical growth abnormalities in children, while adults and children can manifest diverse side effects such as nausea, muscle weakness, joint stiffness, and elevation in blood pressure (hypertension).

Vitamin E is widely proclaimed as being a "safe" vitamin, with little or no risk to the user, even in amounts greatly exceeding the RDA value for adults (12 to 15 I.U.). Yet, reports do appear in the medical literature which suggest that even Vitamin E is not exempt from producing toxic effects if taken in "megavitamin" doses. For example, a report appeared in the *New England Journal of Medicine* (Vol. 289, pages 979–980, 1973) describing muscle weakness and fatigue resulting from taking 800 I.U. per day for one week. When the vitamin was discontinued, these symptoms disappeared. In some patients the symptoms could be seen with 400 I.U. per day. The doctors who made these observations refer to "hypervitaminosis E." When the syndrome is recognized, the subject merely has to stop taking the vitamin in order for the weakness, malaise, and fatigue to disappear. Cramps and diarrhea also have been reported to occur with high doses of vitamin E (*Canadian Medical Association Journal,* Vol. 110, pages 401–406, 1974). Topically applied Vitamin E (in the form of deodorants, vaginal sprays, or cosmetic creams) can cause skin rashes in susceptible individuals.

A potential hazard of vitamin supplementation in children has received little attention. Most vitamin supplements contain colorants and food additives that may produce allergic responses and emotional upset and learning problems. Preparations for children (for example, chewable vitamins) contain relatively large amounts of these additives, although it should be pointed out that the major intake of these additives is from convenience foods and soft drinks rather than vitamin supplements.

Thus, it should be clear to everyone that (1) taking too much of some vitamins can do severe damage, (2) not only should you not self-medicate, but you should not place your health and well-being in the hands of a well-meaning but untrained vitamin salesman. Furthermore, do not fool yourself, or try to fool your physician!

Antivitamins

An intriguing concept that has received increasing scientific attention is that of "antivitamins" (see Glossary). Originally the term was used in connection with the general concept of antimetabolites (substances that interfere with or antagonize normal actions of vital cellular substances). Thus, antivitamins are of two types: (1) substances chemically similar to the vitamins and (2) substances that destroy or decrease the biological effects of a vitamin (see National Academy of Sciences Committee on Food Protection, 1973).

Are these definitions only of theoretical interest? No. Consider Vitamin E. Increased dietary intake of polyenic acids (fatty acids) increases the need for Vitamin E. Also remember: some polyunsaturated "vegetable" oils contain large amounts of Vitamin E. Chemical factors in certain beans cancel the action of Vitamin E in preventing nutritional muscular dystrophy in hens. If one consumes large amounts of Vitamin E, antagonism of Vitamin A action occurs; the opposite may also occur. (Low doses of Vitamin E improve the utilization of Vitamin A, however!)

Nature provides abundant and exotic sources of antivitamins. Antithiamine (B_1) substances have been isolated from carp, crab, mussels, seastars, fish of the salmon genus, and certain Hawaiian fishes! Consumption by man of mussels (Venus mercenaria) frequently found on the Atlantic seaboard can cause complete destruction of thiamine.

The sea is not the only source of antithiamine substances. Blueberries, black currants, red beets, Brussels sprouts, red cabbage, rice bran, and spinach all have inactivated thiamine to one degree or another.

Natural antagonists of riboflavin (B_2), niacin, biotin, pyridoxine, pantothenic acid, vitamins A, and D also have been described. Other examples have been discussed in the section on Vitamins in Relation to Other Substances.

Factors Influencing
Vitamin Potency

The vitamin content of foods is not invulnerable to change and destruction. Storage, processing, and cooking can significantly modify the content of vitamins from that seen in the fresh food. Similarly, pure synthetic vitamins may lose their stated potency by exposure to sunlight or excessive heat, or by merely aging in the container. This is why most quality-controlled brand-name vitamin preparations have expiration dates stamped on their labels. This expiration dating does not imply that the potency of the vitamins is totally and suddenly lost at a certain date. What does happen is a gradual reduction in potency below that approved by the Food and Drug Administration. Thus, a Vitamin C preparation that contains 100 mg tablets of the vitamin may variably lose some of its biological activity depending upon the quality of manufacture and chemical purity, as well as storage conditions. Furthermore, recent studies have shown that the tablets decay into a substance that may produce high blood uric acid levels which may be detected when routine blood tests are performed.

When an expiration date appears on a vitamin preparation, and that date is due, it is the responsibility of either the manufacturer or the retail store to replace the dated item with fresh material. This is analogous to the open dating that is now used widely with dairy products.

V

OTHER
ASPECTS OF
NUTRITION

Water, Energy, Acids, Minerals

We have tried to limit our discussion to vitamins. However, we have to mention that vitamins are only one component of the nutritional requirements of the body. Water, energy (to maintain metabolic processes, physical activity, growth, and body temperature), essential proteins (amino acids), essential fatty acids, and minerals are also necessary to maintain health. Each of these requirements will be only briefly mentioned here, although each deserves a chapter equal in importance to the vitamins. This subject has been reviewed by the National Academy of Sciences, from whose publication on 1974 RDA's we have drawn the facts presented below.

Water. Water accounts for one-half to three-quarters of the body weight. Requirements vary with age, activity, and climate. Water in the body is closely associated with the presence of essential chemicals (electrolytes) such as is found in salt (which is composed of two electrolytes, sodium and chloride). The body has excellent natural mechanisms, such as thirst and the control of sweating and urine production, to maintain a proper water and electrolyte content. Problems arise in normal persons generally only when they are unable to drink as much water as their natural mechanisms tell them to. When a normal person requires a lot of water, such as in a hot climate or with heavy exercise, he must also have enough electrolytes, such as salt. Unfortunately, each year healthy persons die from exposure to heat. Some of these, according to the National Academy of Sciences, are young football players during summer training who die because coaches withhold water. Free access to water is essential whenever sweat losses are likely to be high.

Energy. Energy may be derived from any reasonable combination of carbohydrate, fat, and protein. Alcohol can also serve as an energy source but is toxic in large amounts. Dietary intake patterns in the United States have shifted in this century. Carbohydrates were the principal source of energy in the past, but, at the present time, fats make nearly equal contributions to the energy content of the national diet. The total protein content of the food supply has remained nearly constant at 11 to 12 percent of dietary energy.

Energy requirements vary with age, size, activity, and climate. Pregnant and nursing women have increased energy requirements. Excessive energy intake leads to obesity; in other words, if you eat too much you get fat! Energy intake is usually not well regulated to maintain balance at very low levels of work output, with the result that inactive people put on weight. If you then go on a diet to lose weight, you may not eat enough of the essential nutrients. Diets of less than 1,800 to 2,000 kcal (see Glossary) do not have enough of them unless fats, sugar, and alcohol are more rigidly restricted than is customary in most American households. Persons who drink alcohol may get 5 to 10 percent of their energy this way, and some people get 1,800 kcal or more a day from alcohol. Many Americans get 30 percent or more of their energy from relatively pure sugars, fats, and alcohol, which provide almost no vitamins and minerals.

Proteins and essential amino acids. Dietary protein provides amino acids and nitrogen for making body proteins and other body components. Even after growth has ceased, amino acids and nitrogen are required continuously to replace losses from the breakdown of body tissues, sweat, body secretions and excretions, and skin, nails and hair growth. For adults, eight amino acids are not produced by the body and thus have to be supplied by the diet. These are called "essential" amino acids. From a nutritional viewpoint, the essential amino acids are the most critical components of dietary proteins; after the requirements for these have been met, the additional nitrogen that is required can be provided in a variety of forms. Growth, pregnancy, and lactation require larger protein intakes.

A word of caution: the Federal Trade Commission (FTC) of the U.S. Government has recently acted to caution the American consumer on the use of protein supplements. The FTC's position is that the American diet contains adequate protein intake and that the promiscuous promotion, sale, and use of protein supplements, without a physician's advice, may cause serious medical problems. Thus, certain individuals with poor kidney function may be unable to excrete the high levels of nitrogen compound formed from excessive protein intake. Of course, there is also the economic factor of purchasing these high-priced protein supplements when they are, in fact, not needed.

Essential fatty acids. Two polyunsaturated fatty acids, linoleic acid (see Glossary) and arachidonic acid, are the only fatty acids known to be essential to many animals and human infants. Linoleic acid cannot be produced by animals and must therefore be supplied in the diet. It occurs in high concentrations in various vegetable oils such as corn, cottonseed, peanut, safflower, and soybean, but not in olive or coconut oil. Arachidonic acid can be formed in the body from linoleic acid; it also occurs in small quantities in animal fats.

Essential fatty acid deficiency in experimental animals produces poor growth, skin problems, poor reproductive performance, decreased resistance, and several other problems. Deficiencies have not been reported in humans except in some hospitalized patients maintained exclusively on intravenous feeding for prolonged periods.

Essential fatty acids seem to play a role in the regulation of cholesterol metabolism, especially transport, transformation, and ultimate excretion. Diets high in polyunsaturated fatty acids (including essential fatty acids) have been shown to reduce serum cholesterol in experimental animals and man.

Essential fatty acids are important for maintaining the function and integrity of cellular and subcellular membranes. In addition, essential fatty acids have been shown to be involved in the production of a group of hormonelike substances called prostaglandins, which are important for many body functions.

Studies with both human subjects and animals indicate that to prevent deficiency the essential fatty acids should be 1 to 2 percent of the total calories. This amount in the diet is not difficult to achieve.

Minerals. Many minerals are required for normal growth and for maintenance of health. Some are required in relatively large amounts (100 mg per day or more) and others are needed in amounts no greater than a few micrograms per day (trace elements). Minerals needed in relatively large amounts are calcium, phosphorous, magnesium, sodium, potassium, and chloride. Seventeen trace elements have been shown to have biological functions in animals. While all of these, and probably others, may eventually prove essential for man, there are only a few for which the present state of knowledge allows an evaluation for human nutrition. These are fluorine, chromium, manganese, iron, cobalt, copper, zinc, selenium, molybdenum, and iodine. Nutritional problems associated with deficient intake of iron, fluoride, and iodine are known to exist in the United States; recent evidence suggests some people may not have enough zinc and chromium.

Bones are often considered to be stable parts of the body; it is a surprise to many people to find out that bone is constantly being formed and reabsorbed. In adult man it has been estimated that 700 mg of calcium enter and leave the bones each day. The major inorganic part of bone is a form of calcium phosphate. The calcium in most diets comes from milk and dairy products; in the United States, 85 percent is obtained this way. Phosphorus is present in nearly all foods, and dietary deficiency is not known to occur in man, except that prolonged and excessive use of nonabsorbable antacids can cause too much phosphorous to be removed from the body. This situation is characterized by weakness, loss of appetite, and pain in the bones. A little-known role of phosphorous is that many of the B vitamins are effective only when combined with phosphate in the body.

Vitamin D is required for efficient absorption of calcium. Changes in protein intake can affect the body's use of calcium. It appears that calcium losses can be substantial when the protein intake is high, and if this situation continues for a long period, it could result in considerable loss of body calcium.

Osteoporosis (bone thinning) can occur in middle and later life especially in women, and it had been thought that this process could be slowed by high calcium intake. However, the scientific evidence does not support this, and the RDA (1974) states that there is no longer any reason, provided Vitamin D intake is adequate, to recommend more than 800 mg of calcium per day.

Magnesium is an essential part of many enzyme systems and is important for nerve and muscle activity. Magnesium deficiency occurs in some infants, in alcoholics, and in severe malnutrition. A deficiency leads to tremors and convulsions and sometimes to behavioral changes. Nevertheless, since magnesium occurs in a variety of foods, particularly vegetables, a dietary deficiency of magnesium seems to be rare.

Sodium, potassium, and chloride, which are all of great importance in body function, occur widely in most diets. Deficiencies of sodium may occur with excessive sweating due to exercise, fever, or heat. Whenever more than four quarts of water is necessary to replace sweat loss, extra salt must be provided. Excessive potassium losses may occur with diarrhea, with the use of purgatives, and with diuretic drugs. Chloride losses occur together with sodium losses. Vomiting also depletes chloride.

The 1974 RDA states that two trends may lead to imbalances of trace element nutrition in the future. First, the increasing use of highly refined or fabricated foods substantially reduces the intake of essential trace nutrients. Second, human exposure to environments contaminated with certain heavy metals for which no essential function is known has increased and can be expected to increase further in the future. The consequences for health of these imbalances are little known, but trace elements, like many nutrients, can cause injury at excessive levels of intake.

There are three situations in which iron intake is frequently inadequate: (1) infancy, because of the low iron content of milk and because the amount of iron the infant has at birth is usually not sufficient to meet the needs beyond six months; (2) during the female reproductive period, because of menstrual iron losses; and (3) in pregnancy, because of the demands of the fetus and losses in childbirth. In these cases it is probably necessary to supplement the normal diet with extra iron. However, it is also possible to increase the iron intake by selecting iron-rich foods whenever possible and by including in the diet foods that are known to increase the absorption of iron present in the diet: for example, meat and citrus fruit.

Copper is an essential nutrient for all mammals, but deficiency is rare in man. It occurs in certain cases of malnutrition and certain kidney diseases. It can occur in premature infants fed exclusively on modified cows' milk for two to three months. Copper is widely distributed in foods; the richest sources of dietary copper are nuts, some shellfish, liver, kidney, and raisins. Copper also is found in drinking water, but the amount varies with the type of piping and with the hardness of water. Human milk is far richer in copper than cows' milk.

Iodine is an important part of thyroid hormones. Its deficiency leads to goiter (see Glossary). Although the addition of iodine to salt has greatly reduced goiter in the United States a 1959–1965 survey in Michigan diagnosed goiter in 6.6 percent of 9,000 persons examined. Women of childbearing age had a 15 percent rate of visible goiters. However, it is not clear that these cases were due to a dietary deficiency of iodine. Shellfish is an excellent source of iodine. Most vegetable products are low in iodine. The use of iodized salt is the most efficient way to supplement dietary iodine. However, only slightly more than half of the table salt consumed in the United States is iodized. Salt added to preprocessed foods by the manufacturer usually does not contain iodine, and salt bought in bulk (for example, by schools and restaurant chains) is unlikely to be iodized.

Fluoride is present in small but widely varying concentrations in practically all soils, water supplies, plants and animals. Fluoride is incorporated into the structure of the teeth and is required for resistance to cavities. Its protective effect is particularly evident during infancy and early childhood, but persists through adult life.

Tea is a good source of fluoride. Vegetables vary in fluoride content depending on the soil in which they are grown. Most animal products provide some fluoride, but small fish that are eaten whole, including the bones (such as sardines), provide more fluoride. In many parts of the United States the daily dietary fluoride intake is not sufficient to provide good protection against dental cavities, and therefore fluoridation of the drinking water has become a common way of providing extra fluoride. It is beyond the scope of this book to comment extensively on the merits of this controversial procedure. Proponents point out that it is an effective means of providing the necessary extra fluoride, while opponents feel that the target population (infants and young children) generally drink milk, juices, or soft drinks rather than water, and that many persons who do not need it (and in fact may be harmed by the fluoride if they are on certain antibiotic medications) are unable to avoid taking in the fluoride in the drinking water. They suggest that only the water supply of schools be fluoridated, while infants and younger children should have the fluoride added to their milk.

The importance of zinc in body processes has been largely ignored. Yet there is mounting evidence that zinc deficiencies can produce serious effects on man and animals. Loss of appetite and failure to grow are the principal results of the deficiency, and in certain animal studies, even temporary deficiencies (for example, during fetal development or for periods shortly after birth) can have permanent effects on the animals.

There are wide areas in the United States in which the soil is deficient in available zinc, and the appearance of spontaneous zinc deficiencies has led to zinc enrichment of animal feeds. Serious zinc deficiencies in man, resulting in hypogonadism (small sex glands) and dwarfism, have been found in the Middle East. Although such serious cases probably do not exist in the United States, some deficiencies have recently been described. For example, in some persons increased wound healing and an improved sense of taste, observed as a result of increased zinc intake, suggests that the zinc requirements of these subjects was not fully met by their diet. Studies of apparently healthy children in Denver have revealed that some who were deficient in zinc intake had a poor sense of taste, poor appetite, and poor body growth. Increasing the daily zinc intake produced marked improvement.

The zinc intake should come from a balanced diet containing sufficient animal protein. Meat, liver, eggs, and seafood (particularly oysters) are good sources of available zinc, followed by milk and whole-grain products—whole wheat or rye bread, oatmeal, whole corn.

A number of other trace elements have been reported to be necessary for good health. In general, little is known about their importance in human nutrition, since most of the studies were undertaken on research animals. More details can be obtained from the 1974 Recommended Dietary Allowance, National Academy of Sciences.

VI

CONCLUSIONS

We have surveyed the scientific literature and controversies relating to vitamins. However, this short survey and review cannot be considered complete; there are some topics we have left out: some by oversight and some intentionally. Nevertheless our hope is that the reader now has a better understanding of vitamins and can make a more logical choice regarding vitamin supplementation.

The word "vitamin" suggests vigorous health; it sounds so much more positive than the word "drug"! A common approach to vitamins is "if a little bit is good, a lot will be better, and enormous quantities still better." We wish to emphasize that taking large doses of vitamins means that the "vitamin" becomes a "drug." This implies that the body must work hard to get rid of this excess drug, that the drug may interact (in some cases adversely) with other substances, that some toxic ("overdose") problems may occur, and that dependency states may be created. These have been discussed in the book.

However, the fact remains that supplementary vitamins are of very great value for certain persons in certain situations: the elderly, those on low-calorie reducing diets, those taking certain medications (such as oral contraceptives, anti-epilepsy drugs, mineral oil for constipation), pregnant women, infants who are not breast-fed, and several others.

In the final analysis, each person is free to decide for himself or herself or for his or her family. Some persons may feel better and have more energy when taking vitamin supplements, even when no deficiencies can be demonstrated. This may involve the placebo effect we have discussed. Others may fall outside the "statistical norm" and actually require more of certain vitamins than the RDA. It is often costly and difficult to determine blood and tissue levels of vitamins to decide if there is a true deficiency, and some persons may opt to be on the safe side by taking vitamin supplements. To these individuals, we only suggest that they consider the possible adverse or toxic effects of large doses of vitamins and take only as much as is considered safe. This book should help in making that decision.

We do not wish to offer medical advice. When we began to write this book, we may have had personal biases and attitudes toward vitamin supplementation and good health. Now that we have completed our survey of the field, we realize that some of our previous attitudes were not based on credible scientific evidence. We have changed these attitudes. Perhaps your views and opinions have been changed similarly by the facts and discussion presented here. As an individual, you may change your opinion again as other scientific evidence convinces you to do so.

APPENDICES

Primary Sources

What Is a Vitamin?

Coldsmith, D. Vitamins—the great American rip-off. *Mod. Med.* Mar. 15, 1975, p. 121.

Folkers, K. Survey on the vitamin aspects of coenzyme Q. *Int. Z. Vitaminforsch.* 39:334, 1969.

Morton, R. The vitamin concept. In: *Vitamins and Hormones* 32: 155, 1974. Academic Press, New York, 1974.

Vitamins and Nutrition

Butterworth, C. Correcting malnutrition: practical therapeutic approaches. *Mod. Med.* Nov. 30, 1970, p. 97.

Crosby, W. Can a vegetarian be well nourished? *JAMA* 233: 898,1975.

Goodhart, R. Vitamin therapy today. *Med. Clin. N.A.* Sept. 1956, p. 1473.

Heenan, J. Myths of vitamins. *FDA Consumer* 544:192, 1974.

Nesheim, R. Nutrient changes in food processing: a current review. *Fed. Proc.* 33:2267, 1974.

Recommended Dietary Allowances

Arnaud, S., Stickler, G. Recent developments in Vitamin D research. *Clin. Ped.* 13:444, 1974.

Goldstein, B., Buckley, R., Cardenas, R., and Balchum, O. Ozone and Vitamin E. *Science* 169:605, 1970.

Harper, A. Those pesky RDAs. *Nutr. Today* 9:15, 1974.

National Acad. Sciences (National Research Council). *Recommended Dietary Allowances.* Eighth Edition, 1974, Washington, D.C.

Recommended dietary allowances. *Dairy Council Digest* 45:13, 1974.

Selander, H., Nilsson, J. Vitamin E and air pollution. *Acta Pharmaceut. Suecica* 9:125, 1972.

Tappel, A. Vitamin E. *Nutr. Today* July/Aug. 1973, p. 4.

Williams, R. *Biochemical Individuality.* John Wiley & Sons, New York, 1956.

――――. *You Are Extraordinary.* Random House, New York, 1967.

Vitamin C and the Common Cold

Anderson, T. Large-scale trials of Vitamin C in the prevention and treatment of colds. *Acta Vitaminol. Enzymol.* 28:99, 1974.

――――. Vitamin C and the common cold. Letter to the editor. *Can. Med. Assoc. J.* 108:133, 1973.

Anderson, T., Beaton, G., Corey, P., and Spero, L. Winter Illness and Vitamin C: the effect of relatively low doses. *Can. Med. Assoc. J.* 112:823, 1975.

Anderson, T., Reid, D., and Beaton, G. Vitamin C and the common cold: a double-blind trail. *Can. Med. Assoc. J.* 107:503, 1972.

Anderson, T., Suranyi, G., Beaton, G. The effect on winter illness of large doses of Vitamin C. *Can. Med. Assoc. J.* 111:31, 1974.

Bouhuys, A. Colds and antihistamine effect of Vitamin C. *N. Eng. J. Med.* 290:633, 1974.

Burr, M. Factors influencing the metabolic availability of ascorbic acid. *Clin. Pharmacol. & Therapeut.* 18:238, 1975.

Coulehan, J., Reisinger, K., Rodgers, K., and Bradley, D. Vitamin C prophylaxis in a boarding school. *N. Eng. J. Med.* 290:6, 1974.

De Chatelet, L., McCall, C., Cooper, M., and Shirley, P. Ascorbic acid levels in phagocytic cells. *Proc. Soc. Exp. Biol. and Med.* 145:1170, 1974.

Dykes, M., and Meier, P. Ascorbic acid and the common cold. *JAMA* 231:1073, 1975.

Herbert, V. Vitamin C. Letters to the Editor, *Nutr. Today* 10:29, 1975.

Hodges, R. The effect of stress on ascorbic acid metabolism in man. *Nutr. Today* 5:11, 1970.

Karlowski, T., Chalmers, T., Frenkel, L., Kapikian, A., Lewis, T., and Lynch, J. Ascorbic acid for the common cold. A Prophylactic and therapeutic trial. *JAMA* 231:1038, 1975.

Loh, H., Odumosu, A., and Wilson, C. Sex and ascorbic acid metabolism. *Clin. Pharmacol. and Ther.* 16:390, 1973.

Masek, J., Hruba, F., Neradilova, M., Hejda, S. The role of Vitamin C in the treatment of acute infections of the upper respiratory pathways. *Acta Vitaminol. Enzymol. (Milano)* 28:85, 1974.

Pauling, L. Early evidence about Vitamin C and the common cold. *J. Orthomol. Psych.* 3:139, 1974.

_____. Evolution and the need for ascorbic acid: *Proc. Nat. Acad. Sci.* 64:1643, 1970.

_____. *Vitamin C and The Common Cold.* W. H. Freeman and Co., San Francisco, 1970.

Ritzel, G. Critical evaluation of Vitamin C as a prophylactic and therapeutic agent in colds. *Helvet. Med. Acta.* 28:63, 1961.

Roine, P., Koivula, L., Pekkarinen, M., Rissanen, A. Vitamin C intake and plasma level among aged people in Finland. *Int. J. Vit. Nutr. Res.* 44:95, 1974.

Schwartz, A., Togo, Y., Hornick, R., Tominaga, S., and Gleckman, R. Evaluation of efficacy of ascorbic acid in prophylaxis of induced rhinovirus-44 infection in man. *J. Infect. Dis.* 128:500, 1973.

Tyrrell, D. Vitamin C and the common cold. *Prescribers' J.* 14:21, 1974.

Stone, I. *The Healing Factor.* Grosset & Dunlap, New York, 1972.

Vitamin C and the common cold. *The Medical Letter* 16:85, 1974.

Wilson, C. The common cold and Vitamin C: prophylactic, therapeutic, metabolic, and functional aspects. *Acta Vitaminol. Enzymol. (Milano)* 28:96, 1974.

_____. Colds, ascorbic acid metabolism, and Vitamin C. *J. Clin. Pharmacol.* 15:570, 1975.

_____. Vitamin C: tissue saturation, metabolism, and desaturation. *Practitioner* 212:481, 1974.

Wilson, C., Loh, H. Foster, F. The beneficial effect of Vitamin C on the common cold. *Eur. J. Clin. Pharmacol.* 6:26, 1973.

_____. Common cold symptomatology and Vitamin C. *Eur. J. Clin. Pharmacol.* 6:196, 1973.

Wilson, C. and Loh, H. Common cold and Vitamin C. *Lancet* 1:638, 1973.

————. Vitamin C metabolism and the common cold. *Eur. J. Clin. Pharmacol.* 7:421, 1974.

Zuskin, E., Lewis, A., and Bouhuys, A. Inhibition of histamine-induced airway constriction by ascorbic acid. *J. Allergy Clin. Immunol.* 51:218, 1973.

Vitamin E and the Heart

Anderson, T., Reid, D. A double-blind trial of Vitamin E in angina pectoris. *Amer. J. Nutr.* 27:1174, 1974.

DeLiz, A. Administration of massive doses of Vitamin E to diabetic schizophrenic patients. *J. Orthomol. Psych.* 4:85, 1975.

Goldstein, B., Buckley, R., Cardenas, R., and Balchum, O. Ozone and Vitamin E. *Science* 169:605, 1970.

Helwing, H., Hochrein, B. Vitamin E in der Behandlung der Digitalis-intoxikation. *Arzneimettel-Forschung* 21:335, 1971.

Hodges, R. Vitamin E, a review. *NUTRAH* 1:1, 1972 (a publication of the American Heart Association).

Olson, R. Vitamin E and its relation to heart disease. *Circul.* 48:179, 1973.

Pinckney, E. The potential toxicity of excessive polyunsaturates. *Am. Heart J.* 85:723, 1973.

Shute, W. and Taub, H. *Vitamin E For Ailing and Healthy Hearts.* Pyramid House, New York, 1969.

Vitamin E—miracle or myth? *FDA Consumer* 584:264, 1964.

Vogelsang, A. Twenty-four years using a-tocopherol in degenerative cardiovascular disease. *Angiol.* 21:275, 1970.

Weiss, P., Bianchine, J. The effect on serum tocopherol levels of drug-induced decrease in serum lipids. *Am. J. Med. Sci.* 258:275, 1969.

Williams, H., Fenna, D., MacBeth, R. Occlusion benefits from Vitamin E. *Surg. Gynec. Obstet.* 133:662, 1971.

Vitamin E and Blood Disorders

Ames, S. Isomers of alpha-tocopherol acetate and their biological activity. *Lipids* 6:281, 1971.

Bieri, J. Gamma tocopherol: metabolism, biological activity and significance in human Vitamin E nutrition. *Am. J. Clin. Nutr.* 27:980, 1974.

Bunnell, R., DeRitter, E., and Rubin, S. Effect of feeding polyunsaturated fatty acids with a low Vitamin E diet on blood levels of tocopherol in men performing hard physical labor. *Am. J. Clin. Nutr.* 28:706, 1975.

Chow, C. Distribution of tocopherols in human plasma and red blood cells. *Amer. J. Clin. Nutr.* 28:756, 1975.

Collected Reprints 1963–1967. Committee on Nutrition. American Academy of Pediatrics, Evanston, Ill., 1968.

Green, J. Vitamin E and the biological antioxidant theory. *Ann. N. Y. Acad. Sci.* 203:29, 1972.

Horwitt, M., Harvey, C., Dahm, C., and Searcy, M. Relationship between tocopherol and serum lipid levels for determination of nutritional adequacy. *Ann. N. Y. Acad. of Sci.* 203:223, 1972.

Skinner, W., Johnson, H., Ellis, M., Parkhurst, R. Relationship between antioxidant and antihemolytic activities of Vitamin E derivatives, In Vitro. *J. Pharmaceut. Sci.* 60:643, 1971.

Tappel, A. Vitamin E. *Nutrition Today* July/Aug. 1973, p. 4.

Weiss, P., Biachine, J. The effect on serum tocopherol levels of drug-induced decrease in serum lipids. *Am. J. Med. Sci.* 258:275, 1969.

Williams, H., Fenna, D., MacBeth, R. Occlusion benefits from Vitamin E. *Surg. Gynec. Obstet.* 133:662, 1971.

Williams, M., Shott, R., O'Neal, P., and Oski, F. Role of dietary iron and fat on Vitamin E deficiency anemia of infancy. *N. Eng. J. Med.* 292:887, 1975.

Vitamin E, Human Fertility, and Sexuality

Myths of Vitamins. *FDA Consumer,* DHEW Publication No. (FDA) 74–2053, U.S. Government Printing Office: 1974 544–192/78.

Vitamin D—Necessary but to Be Used with Caution

Arnaud, S., Stickler, G. Recent developments in Vitamin D research. *Clin. Ped.* 13:444, 1974.

Collected Reprints 1963–1967. Committee on Nutrition. American Academy of Pediatrics, Evanston, Ill., 1968.

DeLuca, H. Vitamin D: the vitamin and the hormone. *Fed. Proc.* 33:2211, 1974.

Hazards of Overuse of Vitamin D. A statement of the Food and Nutrition Board, National Research Council, National Academy of Sciences, Washington, D.C., Nov. 1974.

Kodicek, E. The story of Vitamin D; from vitamin to hormone. *Lancet* Mar. 2, 1974, p. 325.

Kolata, G. Vitamin D: investigations of a new steroid hormone. *Science* 187:635, 1975.

New regulations on Vitamins A and D. *FDA Consumer* 544:189, 1974.

Vitamin D and Heart Attack

Linden, V. Vitamin D and myocardial infarction. *Br. Med. J.* 3: 647, 1974.

Natural versus Synthetic Vitamins

Ames, S. Isomers of alpha-tocopherol acetate and their biological activity. *Lipids* 6:281, 1971.

Kamil, A. How natural are those "natural" vitamins? *J. Nutra. Educ.* 4:92, 1972.

McGilveray, I. Some factors affecting bioavailability. *Int. J. Clin. Pharmacol* 11:340, 1975.

Myths of Vitamins. *FDA Consumer*, DHEW Publication No. (FDA) 74–2053, U.S. Government Printing Office: 1974 544–192/78.

Nesheim, R. Nutrient changes in food processing: a current review. *Fed. Proc.* 33:2267, 1974.

Nilsson, J. Studies of tocopherols and related chromanols. *Acta Pharmaceut. Suecica.* 6:1, 1969.

Orthomolecular Medicine and Megavitamin Therapy

Bryan, P. Keeping prescription drugs safe and effective. *Am. Family Physician* 10:189, 1974.

Butterworth, C. Vitamins, multivitamins, megavitamins, and orthomolecular psychiatry. *Hosp. Formul. Manag.* 10:8, 1975.

Chien, L., Krumdieck, C., Scott, Jr., C., Butterworth, C. Harmful effect of megadoses of vitamins. *Am. J. Clin. Nutr.* 28:51, 1975.

DeLiz, A. Administration of massive doses of Vitamin E to diabetic schizophrenic patients. *J. Orthmol. Psych.* 4:85, 1975.

Dembicki, E. Megavitamins: pro and con. *J. Psychiatr Nurs.* 11:36, 1973.

Hagler, L. and Herman, R. Oxalate metabolism. *Am. J. Clin. Nutr.* part 1, 26:758, 1973; part 2, 26:882, 1973; part 3, 26:1006, 1973; part 4, 26:1073, 1973.

Hawkins, D. and Pauling, L. *Orthomolecular Psychiatry.* W. H. Freeman and Co., San Francisco, 1973.

Hoffer, A. History of orthomolecular psychiatry. *J. Orthomol. Psych.* 3:223, 1974.

―――. The megavitamin scene. *Lancet,* Oct. 12, 1974, p. 908.

―――. The orthomolecular controversy. *J. Orthomol. Psych.* 3:-164, 1974.

Hoffer, J. The controversy over orthomolecular theory. *J. Orthomol. Psych.* 3:167, 1974.

Jelliffe, D. The megavitamin scene. *Lancet* June 15, 1974, p. 1217.

Jukes, T. Megavitamin therapy. *JAMA* 233:550, 1975.

Leff, D. Megavitamins and mental disease. *Med. World News* Aug. 11, 1975, p. 71

"Maternal Nutrition and the Course of Pregnancy" Committee on Maternal Nutrition, Food, and Nutrition Board, National Research Council. National Academy of Sciences, Washington, D. C., 1970.

Megavitamin therapy in psychiatry. *Dairy Council Dig.* 45:23, 1974.

Megavitamins for schizophrenia? Letters to the Editor, *Medical World News,* p. 31, Nov. 3, 1975.

Page, I. From the pitchman and the put-on, protect us. *Modern Medicine,* Oct. 15, 1975.

Pauling, L. Orthomolecular somatic and psychiatric medicine. *J. Vital Subst. Dis. Civiliz.* 14:1, 1968.

―――. Orthomolecular psychiatry. *Science* 160:265, 1968.

Ross, H. Megavitamins. *J. Orthomol. Psych.* 3:254, 1974.

Silverman, L. Orthomolecular treatment in disturbances involving brain function *J. Orthomol. Psych.* 4:71, 1975.

Williams, R. *Biochemical Individuality.* John Wiley & Sons, New York, 1956.

―――. *You Are Extraordinary.* Random House, New York, 1967.

Pregnancy

Gal, I., and Parkinson, C. Vitamin A and carotenoid levels in pregnancy. *Am. J. Clin. Nutr.* 27:688, 1974.

Heller, S., Salkeld, R., Korner, W. Riboflavin status in pregnancy. *Am. J. Clin. Nutr.* 27:1225, 1974.

————. Vitamin B_6 states in pregnancy. *Am. J. Clin. Nutr.* 26:1339, 1973.

"Maternal Nutrition and the Course of Pregnancy" Committee on Maternal Nutrition, Food and Nutrition Board, National Research Council. National Academy of Sciences, Washington, D.C., 1970.

Nutritional needs during pregnancy. *Dairy Council Dig.* 45: July-Aug, 1974.

Ticca, M., Passetto, N. Le vitamine durante la gravidanza e l'allattamento. *Acta Vitaminol. Enzymol.* (Milano) 14:144, 1974.

Infancy and Childhood

Collected Reprints 1963–1967. Committee on Nutrition. American Academy of Pediatrics, Evanston, Ill. 1968.

Fomon, S. *Infant Nutrition.* W. B. Saunders, Inc., Phil., 1967.

"Maternal Nutrition and the Course of Pregnancy." Committee on Maternal Nutrition, Food and Nutrition Board, National Academy of Sciences, Washington, D.C. 1970.

Sauberlich, H., Carhan, J., Baker, E., Raica, N., Herman, Y. Biochemical assessment of the nutritional states of Vitamin B_6 in the human. *Am. J. Clin. Nutr.* 25:629, 1972.

Ticca, M., Passetto, N. Le vitamine durante la gravidanza e l'allattamento. *Acta Vitaminol. Enzymol. (Milano)* 14:144, 1974.

Aging and Geriatrics

Burr, M. L. Factors influencing the metabolic availability of ascorbic acid. *Clin. Pharmacol. & Therapeut.* 18:238, 1975.

Corless, D., Boucher, B., Beer, M., Gupta, S., and Cohen, R. Vitamin-D status in long-stay geriatric patients. *Lancet* June 28, 1974, p. 1404.

Exton-Smith, A., Scott, D., Eds. *Vitamins in the elderly* (Proceedings of a Symposium at Royal College of Physicians, London), John Wright & Sons, Bristol, 1968.

Griffiths, W. *In:* Exton-Smith A., and Scott, D., Eds. *Vitamins in the elderly* (Proceedings of a symposium at Royal College of Physicians, London). John Wright & Sons, Bristol, 1968.

Harman, D. Prolongation of life: role of free radical reactions in aging. *J. Am. Geriat. Soc.* 17:721, 1969.

Mayer, J. Aging and nutrition. *Geriatrics,* May. 1974.

Nitra, M. Confusional states in relation to vitamin deficiencies in the elderly. *J. Am. Geriat. Soc.* 19:536, 1971.

Nowak, G. Nutrition for the aged. (Literature listing 211 citations in English), National Library of Medicine, U.S. Dept. of Health, Education, and Welfare, Lit. Search No. 74–22. (1972–1974).

Nutrition and the Aged. Nutritional Perspectives No. 6, Mead Johnson Laboratories Lit. 107, Feb. 1975.

Roine, P., Koivula, L., Pekkarinen, M., and Rissanen, A., Vitamin C intake and plasma level among aged people in Finland. *Int. J. Vit. Nutr. Res.* 44:95, 1974.

Watkin, D. Nutritional problems today in the elderly in the United States. *In:* Exton-Smith, A., and Scott, D., Eds. *Vitamins for the Elderly* (Proceedings of a Symposium at the Royal College of Physicians, London). John Wright & Sons, Bristol, 1968.

———. A year of developments in nutrition and aging. *Med. Clin. N.A.* 54:1589, 1970.

Whanger, A. Vitamins and vigor at 65 plus. *Postgrad. Med.* 53:167, 1973.

Brain Function

Adams, P., Wynn, V., and Rose, D. Effect of pyridoxine hydrochloride (Vitamin B_6) upon depression associated with oral contraception. *Lancet* 1:897, 1973.

Anonymous. The relation of malnutrition to brain development and behavior. *Nutr. Today* July-Aug. 1974, p. 12.

Arnaud, S., Stickler, G. Recent developments in Vitamin D research. *Clin. Ped.* 13:444, 1974.

Bach-y-Rita, P. *Brain Mechanisms in Sensory Substitution.* Academic Press, New York, 1972.

Brain Function and Malnutrition: Neuropsychological Methods of Assess-

ment. Eds. Precott, J., Read, M., and Coursin, D. John Wiley & Sons, New York, 1975.

Croft, L. Ascorbic acid status of the drug addict patient. *Am. J. Clin. Nutr.* 26:6, 1974.

Faivre, M., Saif, N., and Barral, C. Accidents de la Vitamine B₁₂. *Lyon Med.* 233:987, 1975.

Kelsall, M. Vitamin B₆ in metabolism of the nervous system. *Ann. N. Y. Acad. Sci.* 166:1, 1969.

Manocha, S. *Malnutrition and Retarded Human Development.* Charles C. Thomas, Springfield, Ill., 1972.

Nitra, M. Confusional states in relation to vitamin deficiencies in the elderly. *J. Am. Geriat. Soc.* 19:536, 1971.

Raine, D. N. Effect of treatment on Tryptophan metabolism in childhood epilepsy. *In: Vitamin B₆ Metabolism of the Nervous System,* Ed. Kelsall, M. Am. N.Y. Acad. Sci. 166:297, 1969.

Reynolds, E. Anticonvulsants, folic acid and epilepsy. *Lancet* June 16, 1973, p. 1376.

Roine, P., Koivula, L., Pekkarinen, M., Rissanen, A. Vitamin C intake and plasma level among aged people in Finland. *Int. J. Vit. Nutr. Res.* 44:95, 1974.

Silverman, L. Orthomolecular treatment in disturbances involving brain function. *J. Orthomol. Psych.* 4:71, 1975.

Winick, M. Nutrition and mental development. *Med. Clin. N.A.* 54:1413, 1970.

Wurtman, R., and Fernstrom, J. Effects of the diet on brain neurotransmitters. *Nutr. Rev.* 32:193, 1974.

Oral Contraceptives

Adams, P., Wynn, V., and Rose, D. Effect of pyridoxine hydrochloride (Vitamin B₆) upon depression associated with oral contraception. *Lancet* 1:897, 1973.

Briggs, M. and Briggs, M. Thiamine status and oral contraceptives. *Contraception* 2:151, 1975.

Brown, R., Rose, D., Leklem, J., Linkswiler, H., and Anand, R. Urinary 4-pyridoxic acid, plasma pyridoxal phosphate, and erythrocyte aminotransferase levels in oral contraceptive users receiving controlled intakes of Vitamin B₆. *Am. J. Clin. Nutr.* 28:10, 1975.

Davis, R., and Smith, B. Pyridoxal, Vitamin B$_{12}$ and folate metabolism in women taking oral contraceptive agents. *S. A. Med. J.* 48:1937, 1974.

Feminins and other vitamin-mineral supplements for women taking oral contraceptives. *Med. Letter* 15:81, 1973.

Harris, A. Vitamins and oral contraceptives. *Lancet* 2:82, 1975.

Horwitt, M., Harvey, C., and Dahm, C. Relationship between levels of blood lipids, Vitamins C, A, and E, serum copper compounds, and urinary excretions of tryptophan metabolites in women taking oral contraceptive therapy. *Am. J. Clin. Nutr.* 28:403, 1975.

Miller, L., Benson, E., Edwards, M., and Young, J. Vitamin B$_6$ metabolism in women using oral contraceptives. *Am. J. Clin. Nutr.* 27:797, 1974.

Prasad, A., Oberleas, D., Lei, K., Moghissi, K., and Stryker, J. Effect of oral contraceptive agents on nutrients: 1. Minerals. *Am. J. Clin. Nutr.* 28:377, 1975.

Prasad, A., Lei, K., Oberleas, D., Moghissi, K., and Stryker, J. Effect of oral contraceptive agents on nutrients: 2. Vitamins. *Am. J. Clin. Nutr.* 28:385, 1975.

Smith, J., Goldsmith, G., and Lawrence, J. Effects of oral contraceptive steroids on vitamin and lipid levels in serum. *Am. J. Clin. Nutr.* 28:371, 1975.

Vitamin-contraceptive interactions: The clinical consequences are still a puzzle. *Hosp. Formul. Manag.* Nov. 3, 1975, p. 552.

Winston, F. Oral contraceptives, pyridoxine and depression. *Am. J. Psych.* 130:1217, 1973.

Wynn, V. Vitamins and oral contraceptive use. *Lancet* Mar. 8, 1975.

Yeung, D., and Chan, P. Effects of a progestogen and a sequential type oral contraceptive on plasma Vitamin A, Vitamin E, cholesterol and triglycerides *Am. J. Clin. Nutr.* 28:686, 1975.

Alcoholism

Hines, J. Hematologic abnormalities involving Vitamin B$_6$ and folate metabolism in alcoholic subjects. *N. Y. Acad. Sci.* 252:316, 1975.

Sprince, H., Parker, C., Smith, G., and Gonzales. L. Protective action of ascorbic acid and sulfur compounds against acetaldehyde toxicity: implications in alcoholism and smoking. *Agents and Actions* 5:164, 1975.

————. Protection against acetaldehyde toxicity by ascorbic acid plus reserpine or atropine. *Fed. Proc.* 34: no. 3, Mar. 1, 1975.

Van Thiel, D., Gavaler, J., and Lester, R. Ethanol inhibition of Vitamin A metabolism in the testes: possible mechanism for sterility in alcoholics. *Science* 186:941, 1974.

Cancer

Black, H. Effects of dietary antioxidants on actinic tumor induction. *Res. Com. Chem. Path. and Pharm.* 7:783, 1974.

Bollag, W. Effects of Vitamin A acid on transplantable and chemically induced tumors. *Cancer Chem. Rep.* 55:53, 1971.

Bollag, W., and Ott, F. Therapy of actinic keratoses and basal cell carcinomas with local application of Vitamin A acid. *Cancer Chem. Rep.* 55:59, 1971.

Carmel, R. Extreme elevation of serum transcobalamin I in patients with metastatic cancer. *N. Eng. J. Med.* 292:282, 1975.

Gailani, S., Ohnuma, T., and Rosen, F. Nutritional approaches to cancer therapy. *In: Cancer Medicine,* Eds. Holland, E. and Frei, III, E., Lea and Febiger, Phil., 1974.

Garb, S. *Cure for Cancer—A National Goal.* Springer Publishing Co. Inc., New York, 1968.

Lane, M., Alfrey, C., Mengel, C., Doherty, M., and Doherty, J. The rapid induction of human riboflavin deficiency with galactoflavin. *J. Clin. Invest.* 43:357, 1964.

Leukemia. Ed., Gunz, F., and Baikie, A., 3rd Ed.. Grune and Stratton, New York, 1974.

Markello, J., Rosen, F., and Regelson, W. Studies on a possible relationship between E deficiency and anemia associated with cancer. *Cancer* 17:203, 1964.

Maugh, T. Vitamin A: potential protection from carcinogens. *Science* 186:1198, 1974.

————. Vitamin B_{12}: after 25 years, the first synthesis. *Science* 179:266, 1973.

Meng, H. Parenteral nutrition: principals, nutrient requirements, and techniques. *Geriatrics* 30:97, 1975.

Nutrition, Diet, and Cancer. *Dairy Council Digest,* 46:25, 1975.

Rivlin, R. Riboflavin and cancer: a review. *Cancer Res.* 33:1977, 1973.

Shils, M. Nutrition and Neoplasia, *In: Modern Nutrition in Health and Disease,* Eds. Goodhart, R., and Shils, M. 5th edition, Lea & Febiger, Philadelphia, 1975.

Smith, A., and Kenyon, D. A unifying concept of carcinogenesis and its therapeutic implications. *Oncology* 27:459, 1973.

Tashima, C. Hypercalcemia in cancer: response to therapy. *Am. Family Physician* 10:189, 1974.

Vitamins in Relation to Other Substances

Afroz, M., Bhothinard, B., Etzkorn, J., Horenstein, S., and McGarry, J. Vitamin C and B_{12}. *JAMA* 232:246, 1975.

Ascorbic acid and cholesterol levels. *Med. World News* June 30, 1975, p. 9.

Bieri, J. Effect of excessive Vitamins C and E on Vitamin A status. *Am. J. Clin. Nutr.* 26:382 1973.

Burr, M. Factors influencing the metabolic availability of ascorbic acid. *Clin. Pharmacol. & Therapeut.* 18:238, 1975.

Croft, L. Ascorbic acid status of the drug addict patient. *Am. J. Clin. Nutr.* 26:1042, 1973.

Davies, J., and Newson, J. Ascorbic acid and cholesterol levels in pastoral peoples in Kenya. *Am. J. Clin. Nutr.* 27:1039, 1974.

Drug Interactions. Eds. Morselli, P., Garattini, S., & Cohen, S. Raven Press, New York, 1974.

Herbert, V., and Jacob, E. Destruction of Vitamin B_{12} by ascorbic acid. *JAMA* 230:241, 1974.

Hines, J. Ascorbic acid and Vitamin B_{12} deficiency. *JAMA* 234:24, 1975.

Hoppner, K., Phillips, W., Murray, T. Data on serum tocopherol levels in a selected group of Canadians. *Canad. J. Physiol. and Pharmacol.* 48:321, 1970.

Houston, J., and Levy, G. Modification of drug biotransformation by Vitamin C in man. *Nature* 255:78, 1975.

Hunter, K., Stern, G. and Laurence, D. Use of levadopa with other drugs. *Lancet* 2:1283, 1970.

Lamy, P. OTC drugs and the ambulant patient: (I) potential

problems in therapy. *Hosp. Formul. Manag.* Sept. 1975, p. 451.

Loh, H., and Wilson, C. The interactions of aspirin and ascorbic acid in normal men. *J. Clin. Pharmacol.* 15:36, 1975.

Miller, L., Benson, E., Edwards, M., and Young, J. Vitamin B_6 metabolism in women using oral contraceptives. *Am. J. Clin. Nutr.* 27:979, 1974.

Peterson, V., Crapok, P., Weininger, J., Ginsberg, H., and Olefsky, J. Quantification of plasma cholesterol and triglyceride levels in hypercholesterolemic subjects receiving ascorbic acid supplements. *Am. J. Clin. Nutr.* 28:584, 1975.

Rhead, W., and Schranzer, G. Risks of long-term ascorbic acid overdosage. *Nutr. Rev.* 29:262, 1971.

Rosenthal, G. Interaction of ascorbic acid and warfarin. *JAMA* 215:1671, 1971.

Sahud, M., Cohen, R. Effect of aspirin ingestion on ascorbic acid levels in rheumatoid arthritis. *Lancet* May 8, 1971, p. 937.

Swidler, G. *Handbook Drug Interactions.* Wiley-Interscience, New York, 1971.

Zannoni, V., and Lynch, M. The role of ascorbic acid in drug metabolism. *Drug Metab. Rev.* 2:57, 1973.

Vitamin Dependency

Darby, W. The rational use of vitamins in medical practice. *Med. Clin. N. A.* 48:1203, 1964.

Placebo Effects

Bush, P. The placebo effect. *J. Am. Pharmaceut. Assoc.* NS14:671, 1974.

Darby, W. The rational use of vitamins in medical practice. *Med. Clin. N. A.* 48:1203, 1964.

Goldstein, A., Aronow, L., and Kalman, S. *Principals of Drug Actions,* Harper & Row, New York, 1968.

Importance of Fundamental Principals in Drug Evaluation. Eds. Tedeschi, D. and Tedeschi, R. Raven Press, New York, 1968.

Pharmacologic Basis of Therapeutics. Eds. Goodman, L. and Gilman, A. Macmillan, New York, 4th Edition, 1970.

Pihl, R., and Altman, J. An experimental analysis of the placebo effect. *J. Clin. Pharmacol.* 2:91, 1971.

The Principals and Practice of Clinical Trials. Eds. Harris, E., and

Fitzgerald, J. E & S Livingstone, Edinburgh, 1970.

Taber, G. *Proving New Drugs,* Geron-X, Los Altos, 1969.

Wolf, S. The pharmacology of placebos. *Pharmacol. Rev.* 11:689, 1959.

Vitamin Toxicity

Anonymous. New regulations on Vitamins A and D. *FDA Consumer* 544:189, 1974.

De Chatelet, L., McCall, C., Cooper, M., and Shirley, P. Ascorbic acid levels in phagocytic cells. *Proc. Soc. Exp. Biol. and Med.* 145:1170, 1974.

Fomon, S., *Infant Nutrition.* W. B. Saunders, Inc., Phil., 1967.

Frame, B., Jackson, C., Reynolds, W., and Umphrey, J. Hypercalcemia and skeletal effects in chronic hypervitaminosis A. *Ann. Int. Med.* 80:44, 1974.

Goodhart, R. Vitamin therapy today. *Med. Clin. N. A.* Sept. 1956, p. 1473.

Hagler, L., and Herman, R. Oxalate metabolism. *Am. J. Clin. Nutr.* part 1. 26:758, 1973.; part 2, 26:882, 1973; part 3, 26:1006, 1973; part 4, 26:1073, 1973.

Hazards of Overuse of Vitamin D A Statement of the Food and Nutrition Board, National Research Council, National Academy of Sciences, Washington, D. C. Nov. 1974.

Marks, J. The fat-soluble vitamins in modern medicine. *In: Vitamins and Hormones* 32:131, 1974, Academic Press, New York, 1974.

Pharmacologic Basis of Therapeutics. Eds. Goodman, L. and Gilman, A. Macmillan, New York, 4th Edition, 1970.

Ruby, L., and Mital, M. Skeletal deformities following chronic hypervitaminosis A. *J. Bone and Jt. Surg.* 56A:1283, 1974.

Russell, R., Boyer, J., Bagheri, S., and Hruban, Z. Hepatic injury from chronic hypervitaminosis A resulting in portal hypertension and ascites. *N. Engl. J. Med.* 291:435, 1974.

Shetty, K., Ajlouni, K., Rosenfeld, P., and Hagen, T. Protracted Vitamin D intoxication. *Arch. Int. Med.* 135:986, 1975.

Factors Influencing Vitamin Potency

Bruno, C., DeCicco, A., and Figliuzzi, E. Additivi alimenti e vitamine. *Acta Vitamin. Enzymol. (Milano)* 28:39, 1974.

Miuccio, C. Variazioni del contenuto di alcune vitamine in vegetali durante la conservazione. *Acta Vitamin. Enzymol. (Milano)* 28:23, 1974.

Miuccio, C., Floridi, S., Fidanza, A., Fratoni, A. Effetti indotti dalla cottura sul contenuto in alcune vitamine di diverse specie di pesci surgelati. *Acta Vitamin. Enzymol. (Milano)* 28:35, 1974.

Nesheim, R. Nutrient changes in food processing: a current review. *Fed. Proc.* 33:2267, 1974.

Quaglia, G., Viola, M., and Fidanza, A. Trattementi termici degli alimenti e vitamine. *Acta Vitamin. Enzymol. (Milano)* 28:39, 1974.

Rubin, S., DeRitter, E., and Johnson, J. Stability of Vitamin C. *Am. Pharmaceut. Assoc. Pharmacy Weekly* Aug. 23, 1975, p. 2.

Tomassi, G. Additivi e contenuto in vitamine degli alimenti. *Acta Vitamin. Enzymol. (Milano)* 28:47, 1974.

Water, Energy, Essential Amino Acids, Essential Fatty Acids, Minerals

Anonymous. Nutrition and athletic performance. *Dairy Council Dig.* 46:7, 1975.

Astrand, P. Nutrition and physical performance. *In: Food, Nutrition, and Health, World Rev. Nutr. and Diet* Ed. Rechcigl, M., Washington, 16:59, 1973. Karger, Basel, 1973.

Damon, G. A primer on dietary minerals. *FDA Consumer* 584:266, 1974.

Goodhart, R. Vitamin therapy today. *Med. Clin. N.A.* Sept. 1956, p. 1473.

Pharmacologic Basis of Therapeutics. Eds. Goodman, L. and Gilman, A. Macmillan, New York, 4th Edition, 1970.

Sandstead, H., Burk, E., Booth, G., Darby, W. Current concepts on trace minerals. *Med. Clin, N.A.* 54:1509, 1970.

Williams, S. *Nutrition and Diet Therapy.* C. V. Mosby Co., St. Louis, 1973.

Legislation

H. R. 6807, 94th Congress, House of Representatives, May 7, 1975.

S. 1692, 94th Congress, United States Senate, May 8, 1975.

Glossary of Common Terms

alpha-tocopherol: Vitamin E; obtained from natural sources or prepared synthetically; light yellow, viscous, odorless, oily liquid.

amines: basic organic compounds derived from ammonia by replacement of hydrogen by organic hydrocarbon radicals.

angina pectoris: a disease marked by brief paroxysmal attacks of chest pain caused by deficient oxygenation of the heart muscle; related to insufficient blood flow in coronary arteries to heart.

antihistamine: compounds used for treating allergic reactions and cold symptoms; they act by antagonizing histamine effects on the body.

antioxidant: a substance that prohibits oxidation or inhibits reactions promoted by oxygen or peroxides.

antivitamin: a substance that makes a vitamin ineffective.

atherosclerosis: condition characterized by the deposition of fatty substance (cholesterol?) in, and hardening of, the inner layer of arteries.

barbiturates: group of substances used as sedatives, hypnotics, and anesthetic drugs.

beriberi: a vitamin-deficiency disease marked by inflammation and degeneration of nerves, digestive system, and heart; caused by a lack of, or inability to assimilate, thiamine.

bioavailability: amount of substance, e.g., vitamins, which can be absorbed from the gastrointestinal tract and made available via the blood stream for action on the cells of the body.

bioflavanoid: a biologically active substance, usually drived from citrus sources; alleged ability to maintain normal capillary permeability.

biotin: colorless, crystalline growth vitamins of B complex found in yeast, liver, and egg yolks.

calcium: the most plentiful body mineral; important for structure and growth of bones and teeth; assists in blood clotting; important for proper functioning of nerves, muscles, and heart; some sources are milk and milk products and leafy greens.

calorie: a measure of energy reported in terms of heat; food contains calories, which means that if the food were burned, it would yield the amount of its calories in heat.

carbohydrate: carbon, oxygen, and hydrogen containing compounds found in sugars, starches, and celluloses; a necessary nutrient which supplies energy.

carcinogen: a substance or agent producing or causing cancer.

carotene: any of several orange or red crystalline organic compounds that occur in the plants and in the fatty tissues of plant-eating animals; convertible to Vitamin A.

cholesterol: a fat or fatlike chemical present in animal cells and body fluids; important in physiological processes; implicated as a factor in atherosclerosis ("hardening of the arteries").

coenzyme: nonprotein compound that forms the active portion of an enzyme system (e.g., Coenzyme A). It occurs in all living cells and is essential to the metabolism of carbohydrates, fats, and some amino acids.

cyanocobalamin: B_{12}; a complex cobalt-containing compound that occurs especially in liver; used in treating blood disorders such as pernicious and related anemias.

digitoxin: drug that is used in the treatment of certain forms of heart failure; chemically related to glycosides.

double blind: an experimental procedure in which neither the subjects nor the experimenters know which are the test and which are control groups during the actual course of the experiments.

dysfunction: impaired or abnormal functioning.

epilepsy: disorders marked by disturbed electrical rhythms of the brain and manifested by convulsive attacks or seizures.

fat: combination of glycerol and fatty acids; basic nutrient providing concentrated source of energy.

folate: folic acid, a crystallin acid ($C_{19}H_{19}N_7O_6$) that is a vitamin of the B complex; used in the treatment of nutritional anemias and sprue.

folic acid: vitamin of the B complex used in the treatment of anemia and sprue.

folicin: folic acid or folate.

glycoside: organic derivatives that contain a steroid group attached to a sugar molecule; usually synonymous with digitalis, a drug used for stimulating the heart.

goiter: an enlargement of thyroid gland; associated with abnormality of iodine metabolism.

hemolytic anemia: anemia caused by destruction of red blood cells and the resulting escape of hemoglobin.

hormone: a specific chemical product of an organ or of certain cells of an organ, transported by the blood or other body fluids, and having a specific regulatory effect upon cells remote from its origin; adrenalin and cortisone are examples of circulating hormones.

hypertension: excessive arterial tension, usually synonymous with high blood pressure.

hypervitaminosis: an abnormal state resulting from excessive intake of one or more vitamins.

intermittent claudication: an occlusive vascular disease of vessels of legs, with pain and tenderness of muscles.

international unit: a quantity of a biological (e.g., a vitamin) that produces a particular biological effect, agreed upon by international standard and accord.

iron: mineral needed in small amounts; vital part of hemoglobin, the red substance of blood which carries oxygen from the lungs to all body tissues; assists the body cells in releasing energy from food; sources are liver, kidney, heart, meats, dry beans, whole-grained and enriched breads and cereals, raisins, dark-green leafy vegetables.

isomers: substances of same composition, molecular weight, and equal in other regards, but which differ in the spatial arrangement of atoms in the molecule.

kcal: kilocalorie (i.e., one thousand small calories)

linoleic acid: a liquid, polyunsaturated, fatty acid found in drying and demi-drying oils; essential in animal nutrition.

lipid: substances that include fats, waxes, phosphatides, cerebrosides; basic building block of important cell features such as membranes.

lipoprotein: a group of proteins consisting of a simple protein molecule combined with a lipid (fat).

macrocytic: an exceptionally large red blood cell occurring chiefly in certain anemias due to lack of folic acid or Vitamin B_{12}.

malnutrition: faulty or inadequate nutrition.

megaloblastic anemia: blood disorder caused by lack of folic acid, or Vitamin E deficiency (in infants).

megavitamin: large dose of vitamins

metabolism: phenomena of synthesizing simple foodstuffs into complex tissue elements (anabolism), and breaking down complex substances into simple ones in the production of energy (catabolism).

mg: milligram; one-thousandth of a gram; 0.000035 ounces.

microgram: one-millionth of a gram.

minerals: simple elemental substances that act as body regulators through incorporation into hormones and enzymes; some minerals (calcium, phosphorous, and magnesium) are part of the body's structure.

MDR: minimum daily requirement; the MDR's of five vitamins and four minerals were amounts suggested for daily consumption to prevent demonstrated signs of deficiency; established by the Food and Drug Administration in 1941 and have become obsolete and have been revised and replaced by the U.S. Recommended Daily Allowances (RDA's).

myocardial: pertaining to the muscular functions of the heart; *m. infarction:* dead or scarred heart muscle due to lack of sufficient blood supply.

niacin: same as nicotinic acid; an acid of the Vitamin B complex; required to prevent pellagra.

nicotinamide: a compound of the Vitamin B complex; constituent of coenzymes; used similarly to nicotinic acid (niacin).

nutrient: an important chemical substance in foods that performs one or more of the following functions: (1) furnishes body fuel needed for energy; (2) provides materials needed for the building or maintenance of body tissues; (3) supplies substances that function in the regulation of body processes.

nutrition: the process by which living organisms obtain and use nutrients from food for the maintenance of their functions, for the growth and repair of tissues, and for reproduction; the science of nutrition includes understanding the composition of foods and knowledge of proper food selection to obtain an adequate diet.

oral contraceptives: chemical substances (usually steroids) which can be taken by mouth for the prevention of pregnancy; also used in treating some menstrual disorders.

orthomolecular medicine: the treatment of disease by changing the amounts in the body of substances that are normally present in the body and are required for the preservation of good health.

oxalate: an insoluble salt or ester of oxalic acid, which is a strong acid.

pantothenic acid: an oily acid compound of the Vitamin B complex found in all living cells.

pellagra: a disease marked by dermatitis, gastrointestinal disorders, and central nervous system symptoms caused by a diet deficient in niacin and protein.

penicillamine: substance related to penicillin which has marked ability to chelate (attach) to copper ion; used in treatment of Wilson's Disease.

pernicious anemia: anemia marked by a progressive decrease in number and increase in size of the red blood cells; pallor, weakness, and gastrointestinal and nervous disturbances are associated with reduced Vitamin B_{12} absorption from the distal end of the small intestines.

peroxidation: state of being completely oxidized.

pharmacokinetics: the study of bodily absorption, distribution, metabolism, and excretion of drugs and substances.

phlebitis: inflammation of a vein.

placebo: an inert, innocuous, biologically inactive substance (e.g., sugar, lactose) used especially in controlled experiments testing the efficacy of another biologically active substance; sometimes prescribed to affect illnesses.

polyunsaturated: more than one unsaturated chemical bond; in nutrition, usually refers to polyunsaturated fat or oils; such substances are found in vegetable oils, margarine.

prophylactic: protecting against or preventing disease.

protein: complex combination of amino acids essential to living cells.

pyridoxine: a crystalline phenolic alcohol of the Vitamin B_6 group found especially in cereals and convertible in the organism into pyridoxal and pyridoxamine.

racemic: compound or mixture composed of equal amounts of forms of the same compound that deflect polarized light to the right (dextro) or left (levo).

RDA: Recommended Dietary Allowances are those amounts of substances published by the Food and Nutrition Board of the National Research Council which are estimated to be needed for the maintenance of good nutrition and health of normal persons living in U. S. under usual living conditions.

renal: relating to or involving the kidneys.

retinol: the principal form of Vitamin A.

riboflavin: Vitamin B_2; a growth-promoting member of the Vitamin B complex; also known as Vitamin G in some sources.

rickets: a childhood disease characterized especially by soft and deformed bones; caused by failure to assimilate and use calcium and phosphorous normally due to inadequate sunlight or Vitamin D.

saturated: saturated fat contains fatty acids with only saturated bonds; a saturated bond is a chemical structure which cannot accept any additional hydrogen. Saturated fats tend to be of animal origin and solid; in general, saturated fats contain a large proportion of saturated fatty acids in their molecular structure.

schizophrenia: a psychotic disorder characterized by loss of contact with the environment and by disintegration of personality; expressed as disorder of feeling, thought, and conduct.

scurvy: a disease marked by spongy gums, loosening of the teeth, and a bleeding into the skin and mucous membranes; caused by a lack of ascorbic acid (Vitamin C).

sodium: important element in the regulation of body water and the acid-base balance; needed for proper muscle function; common source is table salt.

sprue: a chronic disease marked by fatty diarrhea and symptoms of nutritional deficiency.

steroid: important substance found e.g. in male sex hormones, female hormones, and components of certain oral contraceptive preparations.

thiamine: a vitamin of the Vitamin B complex that is essential to normal metabolism and nerve function: Vitamin B_1.

tocopherol: any of several fat-soluble, oily phenolic compounds with varying degrees of antioxidant Vitamin E activity.

toxemia of pregnancy: a condition sometimes seen in pregnancy in which the blood contains poisonous products or toxins. Symptoms include muscle cramps, high blood pressure, retention of body fluids, headache, visual disturbances.

toxicity: state of being poisonous.

tryptophan: a crystalline amino acid that is widely distributed in proteins and is essential to animal life.

unsaturated fatty acids: fatty acids which have one or several double bonds between carbons and can add on more hydrogen when these double bonds are broken and reduced to single bonds; hence they are unsaturated in respect to hydrogen (see also *polyunsaturated*).

USP: United States Pharmacopoeia: a quasi-official monograph containing information about drugs and substances used in human biology. Standards of purity, identity, and action are indicated.

vasodilator: a substance producing dilation of blood vessels.

vitamins: any of various organic substances that are essential in minute quantities to the nutrition of most animals and humans and some plants; act especially as coenzymes and precursors of coenzymes in the regulation of metabolic processes; do not provide energy or serve as building units; are present in natural foodstuffs or sometimes produced in the body (e.g., B_{12}).

Wilson's Disease: a congenital disease characterized by excessive stores of copper in the liver.

RECOMMENDED DAILY DIETARY ALLOWANCES FOR VITAMINS*

	A	D (I.U.)	E	C (mg)	FOLACIN (µg)	NIACIN (mg)	RIBOFLAVIN (mg)	THIAMINE (mg)	B_6 (mg)	B_{12} (µg)
Infants										
0–0.5 years	1,400	400	4	35	50	5	0.4	0.3	0.3	0.3
0.5–1.0	2,000	400	5	35	50	8	0.6	0.5	0.4	0.3
Children										
1–3	2,000	400	7	40	100	9	0.8	0.7	0.6	1.0
4–6	2,500	400	9	40	200	12	1.1	0.9	0.9	1.5
7–10	3,300	400	10	40	300	16	1.2	1.2	1.2	2.0
Males										
11–14	5,000	400	12	45	400	18	1.5	1.4	1.6	3.0
15–18	5,000	400	15	45	400	20	1.8	1.5	1.8	3.0
19–22	5,000	400	15	45	400	20	1.8	1.5	2.0	3.0
23–50	5,000	–	15	45	400	18	1.6	1.4	2.0	3.0
51 +	5,000	–	15	45	400	16	1.5	1.2	2.0	3.0
Females										
11–14	4,000	400	10	45	400	16	1.3	1.2	1.6	3.0
15–18	4,000	400	11	45	400	14	1.4	1.1	2.0	3.0
19–22	4,000	400	12	45	400	14	1.4	1.1	2.0	3.0
23–50	4,000	–	12	45	400	13	1.2	1.0	2.0	3.0
51 +	4,000	–	12	45	400	12	1.1	1.0	2.0	3.0
Pregnant	5,000	400	15	60	800	+2	+0.3	+0.3	2.5	4.0
Lactating	6,000	400	15	60	600	+4	+0.5	+0.3	2.5	4.0

*These RDA values (revised 1973) are those recommended by the Food and Nutrition Board, National Academy of Sciences, National Research Council. See Primary Sources for publication source.

Recent Vitamin Legislation

When we began researching the material for this book, we were aware of potential legislation that would have significant effects on the manufacture, promotion, and sale of vitamins. One such bill was introduced into the U.S. Senate on May 8, 1975. The bill is S. 1692 authored by senators Proxmire and Schweiker. The bill is "to amend the Federal Food, Drug and Cosmetic Act to establish certain limitations respecting the authority of the Secretary of Health, Education, and Welfare to regulate vitamins and minerals under that Act, and for other purposes." Sounds innocent enough? Here are the specific sections relating to vitamins (our emphasis added):

Sec. 411 (a)(1). Except as provided in paragraph 2.

(A) The Secretary (of HEW) *may not establish maximum limits* on the potency of any synthetic or natural vitamin or mineral within a food . . .

(B) The Secretary *may not classify any vitamin or mineral as a drug on the basis of the potency of the vitamin* or mineral or on any other basis *other than the fact that*—

(i) the vitamin . . . is *represented in its labeling* for use in the diagnosis, cure, mitigation, treatment, or prevention of disease in man; or

(ii) a condition (including toxicity) which—

(I) is described in Section 503 (b)(1) and

(II) requires that a drug be dispensed only upon prescription . . .

(C) The Secretary *may not limit the combination or number* of any synthetic or natural (i) vitamin, (ii) mineral, or (iii) other ingredient of food, within a food . . .

Additional sections provide that the Secretary of HEW can specify limits for vitamins, minerals, or ingredients of food for use by children or pregnant or lactating women. (Children are defined as individuals under the age of twelve years.) Extensive descriptions of what constitutes a "food" or "special dietary use" are given, especially as they pertain to vitamins and minerals. Language is given defining the penalties (and nonpenalties) pertaining to "advertising" and "labeling" of foods and foods containing vitamins.

The intent of the bill is clear: Congress is being asked to restrict the FDA or other agencies from requiring restrictive or outright "drug" labeling, or prescription requirements for vitamins and minerals, alone or in combination. Only broad powers will allow HEW to restrict vitamins (and their labels) because of toxicity, or special needs, as in children and pregnancy.

The FDA has now published revised administrative regulations which in effect admits they are giving up their recent efforts to reclassify high potency vitamin preparations as drugs. When the agency first proposed such an idea of a reclassification, they were guided by the principle that any vitamin or mineral preparation containing more than 150 percent of the RDA for each substance should be classified as a drug. It was obvious that their scientific staff was concerned and aware that many so-called supervitamin preparations that could be bought over the counter without prescription could be potentially dangerous (hypervitaminosis). Moreover, the FDA through its advertising surveillance program was aware that some manufacturers were using hard-sell techniques and were misrepresenting or exaggerating claims of efficacy and the diseases and illnesses which could be treated with the supervitamin preparations. Their concern appeared to have credence and broad scientific support.

However, under the new revised regulations published in the May 27, 1975, issue of the *Federal Register,* the FDA has agreed to regulate the supervitamins as food. Preparations containing high doses of Vitamins A and D, because of their well-known toxicity, particularly in children, will continue to be regulated as prescription items. Apparently no one objects to this restriction. Importantly, the new FDA position abandons the original idea that would have limited so-called dietary supplements to 150 percent of the RDA of a single vitamin or mineral. The agency also announced that it will now consider new applications from manufacturers wishing to have their new vitamin mineral combinations approved by the FDA.

In the aftermath of this, which has certainly surprised many observers of the workings of the FDA, the agency still intends to use its authority to rule out certain combinations of vitamins and minerals. Such combinations they observe are now widely marketed in health food stores and are irrational in scope and intent.

These recent events may be hailed as a victory for "freedom of choice" vitamin advocates. Perhaps this is so. On the other hand, the sound scientific evidence which was guiding the FDA on this matter apparently was buried by an avalanche of consumer and industry claims and wishes. Such actions are cited as evidence that in a democracy, government is responsive to the people it governs. Yet, we wonder whether the governed (i.e., consumers) were adequately exposed to both sides of the debate. Hopefully, the fact there will not be any notable restrictions on vitamin potency and labeling practices will not result in an outbreak of hypervitaminosis. If widespread or notable vitamin abuse does occur, we can be assured that restrictive legislation again will be attempted.

Our view is that a thoroughly informed citizenry can and must be the judge of claims and counterclaims. Not to be so informed opens the door for those who either will demand oppressive controls, or who will promote unbridled vitamin hucksterism.

Index

The Authors

Joseph V. Levy, Ph.D. (Associate Professor) and Paul Bach-y-Rita, M.D. (Professor) both hold academic appointments in the School of Medical Sciences, University of the Pacific in San Francisco. Both are former holders of Research Career Development Awards from The National Institutes of Health, U. S. Department of Health, Education and Welfare.

Dr. Levy is director of the Laboratory of Pharmacology and Experimental Therapeutics at the Institutes of Medical Sciences in San Francisco. He has authored more than sixty-five articles in scientific journals and books. Dr. Bach-y-Rita, a former Public Health Physician involved in rural medical and nutritional problems, has written approximately one hundred scientific articles and three books dealing with brain function and neurophysiology.